# Mometrix
## TEST PREPARATION

# Certified Coding Associate Exam
## Secrets Study Guide

# Dear Future Exam Success Story

First of all, **THANK YOU** for purchasing Mometrix study materials!

Second, congratulations! You are one of the few determined test-takers who are committed to doing whatever it takes to excel on your exam. **You have come to the right place.** We developed these study materials with one goal in mind: to deliver you the information you need in a format that's concise and easy to use.

In addition to optimizing your guide for the content of the test, we've outlined our recommended steps for breaking down the preparation process into small, attainable goals so you can make sure you stay on track.

We've also analyzed the entire test-taking process, identifying the most common pitfalls and showing how you can overcome them and be ready for any curveball the test throws you.

Standardized testing is one of the biggest obstacles on your road to success, which only increases the importance of doing well in the high-pressure, high-stakes environment of test day. Your results on this test could have a significant impact on your future, and this guide provides the information and practical advice to help you achieve your full potential on test day.

**Your success is our success**

**We would love to hear from you!** If you would like to share the story of your exam success or if you have any questions or comments in regard to our products, please contact us at **800-673-8175** or **support@mometrix.com**.

Thanks again for your business and we wish you continued success!

Sincerely,
The Mometrix Test Preparation Team

---

**Need more help? Check out our flashcards at:**
**http://MometrixFlashcards.com/CodingAssociate**

---

Copyright © 2024 by Mometrix Media LLC. All rights reserved.
Written and edited by the Mometrix Exam Secrets Test Prep Team
Printed in the United States of America

# Table of Contents

Introduction ........................................................................................................ 1
Secret Key #1 – Plan Big, Study Small ............................................................. 2
Secret Key #2 – Make Your Studying Count .................................................... 3
Secret Key #3 – Practice the Right Way ........................................................... 4
Secret Key #4 – Pace Yourself .......................................................................... 6
Secret Key #5 – Have a Plan for Guessing ....................................................... 7
Test-Taking Strategies ..................................................................................... 10
Clinical Classification Systems ...................................................................... 15
    Interpreting Healthcare Data for Code Assignment ..................................... 15
    Incorporating Clinical Vocabularies and Terminologies ............................. 16
    Abstracting Information from Medical Records ........................................... 17
    Consulting Reference Materials .................................................................. 18
    Applying Coding Guidelines ....................................................................... 19
    Assigning Codes .......................................................................................... 27
    Code Sequencing According to Healthcare Setting ..................................... 32
    Determining Evaluation and Management (E/M) Level ............................. 33
    Using Appropriate Modifiers ....................................................................... 36
Reimbursement Methodologies ...................................................................... 38
    Code Sequencing and Payer Specific Guidelines ........................................ 38
    DRG and APC Methodologies .................................................................... 39
    NCCI Edits .................................................................................................. 42
    Coverage Determinations ............................................................................ 43
    Claim Forms ................................................................................................ 44
    Communicating with Financial Departments ............................................. 45
    Claim Denials .............................................................................................. 46
    Communicating Physicians to Clarify Documentation ............................... 48
    Hierarchical Condition Categories (HCCs) and Risk Adjustment .............. 49
    Bundling and Unbundling ........................................................................... 49
Health Records and Data Content .................................................................. 51
    Retrieving Medical Records ........................................................................ 51
    Analyzing Medical Records ........................................................................ 52
    Data Abstraction ......................................................................................... 53
    Patient-Specific Documentation from Other Sources ................................. 54
    Master Patient Index ................................................................................... 55
    Health Data Standards ................................................................................ 56
    Interpreting Reports for Data Analysis ....................................................... 57
    Components of the Medical Record ............................................................ 58
Compliance ....................................................................................................... 60
    Documentation ............................................................................................ 60
    Ethical Coding ............................................................................................. 61

| | |
|---|---|
| Physician Queries | 61 |
| Coding Changes | 64 |
| Educating Providers on Compliant Coding | 66 |
| External Audits | 67 |

## Information Technologies — 69

| | |
|---|---|
| Navigating Throughout the EHR | 69 |
| Encoding and Grouping Software | 70 |
| Practice Management and HIM System | 70 |
| Computer Assisted Coding Software | 71 |

## Confidentiality & Privacy — 73

| | |
|---|---|
| Ensuring Patient Confidentiality | 73 |
| Recognizing and Reporting Privacy Issues or Violations | 75 |
| Maintaining a Secure Work Environment | 76 |
| Minimum Necessary Documentation and Release of Information | 77 |
| Protecting Electronic Documentation | 79 |
| Record Retention and Destruction | 80 |
| Information Blocking | 82 |

## CCA Practice Test #1 — 83

## Answer Key and Explanations for Test #1 — 107

## CCA Practice Test #2 — 131

## Answer Key and Explanations for Test #2 — 149

## How to Overcome Test Anxiety — 167

## Additional Bonus Material — 173

# Introduction

**Thank you for purchasing this resource**! You have made the choice to prepare yourself for a test that could have a huge impact on your future, and this guide is designed to help you be fully ready for test day. Obviously, it's important to have a solid understanding of the test material, but you also need to be prepared for the unique environment and stressors of the test, so that you can perform to the best of your abilities.

For this purpose, the first section that appears in this guide is the **Secret Keys**. We've devoted countless hours to meticulously researching what works and what doesn't, and we've boiled down our findings to the five most impactful steps you can take to improve your performance on the test. We start at the beginning with study planning and move through the preparation process, all the way to the testing strategies that will help you get the most out of what you know when you're finally sitting in front of the test.

We recommend that you start preparing for your test as far in advance as possible. However, if you've bought this guide as a last-minute study resource and only have a few days before your test, we recommend that you skip over the first two Secret Keys since they address a long-term study plan.

If you struggle with **test anxiety**, we strongly encourage you to check out our recommendations for how you can overcome it. Test anxiety is a formidable foe, but it can be beaten, and we want to make sure you have the tools you need to defeat it.

# Secret Key #1 – Plan Big, Study Small

There's a lot riding on your performance. If you want to ace this test, you're going to need to keep your skills sharp and the material fresh in your mind. You need a plan that lets you review everything you need to know while still fitting in your schedule. We'll break this strategy down into three categories.

## Information Organization

Start with the information you already have: the official test outline. From this, you can make a complete list of all the concepts you need to cover before the test. Organize these concepts into groups that can be studied together, and create a list of any related vocabulary you need to learn so you can brush up on any difficult terms. You'll want to keep this vocabulary list handy once you actually start studying since you may need to add to it along the way.

## Time Management

Once you have your set of study concepts, decide how to spread them out over the time you have left before the test. Break your study plan into small, clear goals so you have a manageable task for each day and know exactly what you're doing. Then just focus on one small step at a time. When you manage your time this way, you don't need to spend hours at a time studying. Studying a small block of content for a short period each day helps you retain information better and avoid stressing over how much you have left to do. You can relax knowing that you have a plan to cover everything in time. In order for this strategy to be effective though, you have to start studying early and stick to your schedule. Avoid the exhaustion and futility that comes from last-minute cramming!

## Study Environment

The environment you study in has a big impact on your learning. Studying in a coffee shop, while probably more enjoyable, is not likely to be as fruitful as studying in a quiet room. It's important to keep distractions to a minimum. You're only planning to study for a short block of time, so make the most of it. Don't pause to check your phone or get up to find a snack. It's also important to **avoid multitasking**. Research has consistently shown that multitasking will make your studying dramatically less effective. Your study area should also be comfortable and well-lit so you don't have the distraction of straining your eyes or sitting on an uncomfortable chair.

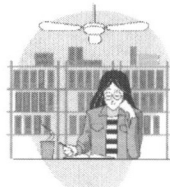

The time of day you study is also important. You want to be rested and alert. Don't wait until just before bedtime. Study when you'll be most likely to comprehend and remember. Even better, if you know what time of day your test will be, set that time aside for study. That way your brain will be used to working on that subject at that specific time and you'll have a better chance of recalling information.

Finally, it can be helpful to team up with others who are studying for the same test. Your actual studying should be done in as isolated an environment as possible, but the work of organizing the information and setting up the study plan can be divided up. In between study sessions, you can discuss with your teammates the concepts that you're all studying and quiz each other on the details. Just be sure that your teammates are as serious about the test as you are. If you find that your study time is being replaced with social time, you might need to find a new team.

# Secret Key #2 – Make Your Studying Count

You're devoting a lot of time and effort to preparing for this test, so you want to be absolutely certain it will pay off. This means doing more than just reading the content and hoping you can remember it on test day. It's important to make every minute of study count. There are two main areas you can focus on to make your studying count.

## Retention

It doesn't matter how much time you study if you can't remember the material. You need to make sure you are retaining the concepts. To check your retention of the information you're learning, try recalling it at later times with minimal prompting. Try carrying around flashcards and glance at one or two from time to time or ask a friend who's also studying for the test to quiz you.

To enhance your retention, look for ways to put the information into practice so that you can apply it rather than simply recalling it. If you're using the information in practical ways, it will be much easier to remember. Similarly, it helps to solidify a concept in your mind if you're not only reading it to yourself but also explaining it to someone else. Ask a friend to let you teach them about a concept you're a little shaky on (or speak aloud to an imaginary audience if necessary). As you try to summarize, define, give examples, and answer your friend's questions, you'll understand the concepts better and they will stay with you longer. Finally, step back for a big picture view and ask yourself how each piece of information fits with the whole subject. When you link the different concepts together and see them working together as a whole, it's easier to remember the individual components.

Finally, practice showing your work on any multi-step problems, even if you're just studying. Writing out each step you take to solve a problem will help solidify the process in your mind, and you'll be more likely to remember it during the test.

## Modality

*Modality* simply refers to the means or method by which you study. Choosing a study modality that fits your own individual learning style is crucial. No two people learn best in exactly the same way, so it's important to know your strengths and use them to your advantage.

For example, if you learn best by visualization, focus on visualizing a concept in your mind and draw an image or a diagram. Try color-coding your notes, illustrating them, or creating symbols that will trigger your mind to recall a learned concept. If you learn best by hearing or discussing information, find a study partner who learns the same way or read aloud to yourself. Think about how to put the information in your own words. Imagine that you are giving a lecture on the topic and record yourself so you can listen to it later.

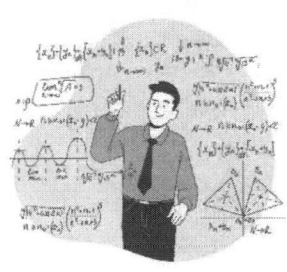

For any learning style, flashcards can be helpful. Organize the information so you can take advantage of spare moments to review. Underline key words or phrases. Use different colors for different categories. Mnemonic devices (such as creating a short list in which every item starts with the same letter) can also help with retention. Find what works best for you and use it to store the information in your mind most effectively and easily.

# Secret Key #3 – Practice the Right Way

Your success on test day depends not only on how many hours you put into preparing, but also on whether you prepared the right way. It's good to check along the way to see if your studying is paying off. One of the most effective ways to do this is by taking practice tests to evaluate your progress. Practice tests are useful because they show exactly where you need to improve. Every time you take a practice test, pay special attention to these three groups of questions:

- The questions you got wrong
- The questions you had to guess on, even if you guessed right
- The questions you found difficult or slow to work through

This will show you exactly what your weak areas are, and where you need to devote more study time. Ask yourself why each of these questions gave you trouble. Was it because you didn't understand the material? Was it because you didn't remember the vocabulary? Do you need more repetitions on this type of question to build speed and confidence? Dig into those questions and figure out how you can strengthen your weak areas as you go back to review the material.

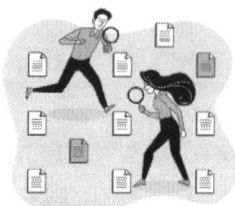
Additionally, many practice tests have a section explaining the answer choices. It can be tempting to read the explanation and think that you now have a good understanding of the concept. However, an explanation likely only covers part of the question's broader context. Even if the explanation makes perfect sense, **go back and investigate** every concept related to the question until you're positive you have a thorough understanding.

As you go along, keep in mind that the practice test is just that: practice. Memorizing these questions and answers will not be very helpful on the actual test because it is unlikely to have any of the same exact questions. If you only know the right answers to the sample questions, you won't be prepared for the real thing. **Study the concepts** until you understand them fully, and then you'll be able to answer any question that shows up on the test.

It's important to wait on the practice tests until you're ready. If you take a test on your first day of study, you may be overwhelmed by the amount of material covered and how much you need to learn. Work up to it gradually.

On test day, you'll need to be prepared for answering questions, managing your time, and using the test-taking strategies you've learned. It's a lot to balance, like a mental marathon that will have a big impact on your future. Like training for a marathon, you'll need to start slowly and work your way up. When test day arrives, you'll be ready.

Start with the strategies you've read in the first two Secret Keys—plan your course and study in the way that works best for you. If you have time, consider using multiple study resources to get different approaches to the same concepts. It can be helpful to see difficult concepts from more than one angle. Then find a good source for practice tests. Many times, the test website will suggest potential study resources or provide sample tests.

# Practice Test Strategy

If you're able to find at least three practice tests, we recommend this strategy:

### UNTIMED AND OPEN-BOOK PRACTICE

Take the first test with no time constraints and with your notes and study guide handy. Take your time and focus on applying the strategies you've learned.

### TIMED AND OPEN-BOOK PRACTICE

Take the second practice test open-book as well, but set a timer and practice pacing yourself to finish in time.

### TIMED AND CLOSED-BOOK PRACTICE

Take any other practice tests as if it were test day. Set a timer and put away your study materials. Sit at a table or desk in a quiet room, imagine yourself at the testing center, and answer questions as quickly and accurately as possible.

Keep repeating timed and closed-book tests on a regular basis until you run out of practice tests or it's time for the actual test. Your mind will be ready for the schedule and stress of test day, and you'll be able to focus on recalling the material you've learned.

# Secret Key #4 – Pace Yourself

Once you're fully prepared for the material on the test, your biggest challenge on test day will be managing your time. Just knowing that the clock is ticking can make you panic even if you have plenty of time left. Work on pacing yourself so you can build confidence against the time constraints of the exam. Pacing is a difficult skill to master, especially in a high-pressure environment, so **practice is vital**.

Set time expectations for your pace based on how much time is available. For example, if a section has 60 questions and the time limit is 30 minutes, you know you have to average 30 seconds or less per question in order to answer them all. Although 30 seconds is the hard limit, set 25 seconds per question as your goal, so you reserve extra time to spend on harder questions. When you budget extra time for the harder questions, you no longer have any reason to stress when those questions take longer to answer.

Don't let this time expectation distract you from working through the test at a calm, steady pace, but keep it in mind so you don't spend too much time on any one question. Recognize that taking extra time on one question you don't understand may keep you from answering two that you do understand later in the test. If your time limit for a question is up and you're still not sure of the answer, mark it and move on, and come back to it later if the time and the test format allow. If the testing format doesn't allow you to return to earlier questions, just make an educated guess; then put it out of your mind and move on.

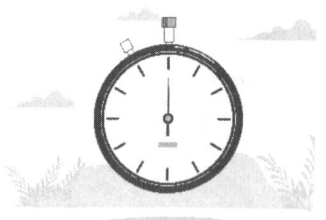

On the easier questions, be careful not to rush. It may seem wise to hurry through them so you have more time for the challenging ones, but it's not worth missing one if you know the concept and just didn't take the time to read the question fully. Work efficiently but make sure you understand the question and have looked at all of the answer choices, since more than one may seem right at first.

Even if you're paying attention to the time, you may find yourself a little behind at some point. You should speed up to get back on track, but do so wisely. Don't panic; just take a few seconds less on each question until you're caught up. Don't guess without thinking, but do look through the answer choices and eliminate any you know are wrong. If you can get down to two choices, it is often worthwhile to guess from those. Once you've chosen an answer, move on and don't dwell on any that you skipped or had to hurry through. If a question was taking too long, chances are it was one of the harder ones, so you weren't as likely to get it right anyway.

On the other hand, if you find yourself getting ahead of schedule, it may be beneficial to slow down a little. The more quickly you work, the more likely you are to make a careless mistake that will affect your score. You've budgeted time for each question, so don't be afraid to spend that time. Practice an efficient but careful pace to get the most out of the time you have.

# Secret Key #5 – Have a Plan for Guessing

When you're taking the test, you may find yourself stuck on a question. Some of the answer choices seem better than others, but you don't see the one answer choice that is obviously correct. What do you do?

The scenario described above is very common, yet most test takers have not effectively prepared for it. Developing and practicing a plan for guessing may be one of the single most effective uses of your time as you get ready for the exam.

In developing your plan for guessing, there are three questions to address:

- When should you start the guessing process?
- How should you narrow down the choices?
- Which answer should you choose?

## When to Start the Guessing Process

Unless your plan for guessing is to select C every time (which, despite its merits, is not what we recommend), you need to leave yourself enough time to apply your answer elimination strategies. Since you have a limited amount of time for each question, that means that if you're going to give yourself the best shot at guessing correctly, you have to decide quickly whether or not you will guess.

Of course, the best-case scenario is that you don't have to guess at all, so first, see if you can answer the question based on your knowledge of the subject and basic reasoning skills. Focus on the key words in the question and try to jog your memory of related topics. Give yourself a chance to bring the knowledge to mind, but once you realize that you don't have (or you can't access) the knowledge you need to answer the question, it's time to start the guessing process.

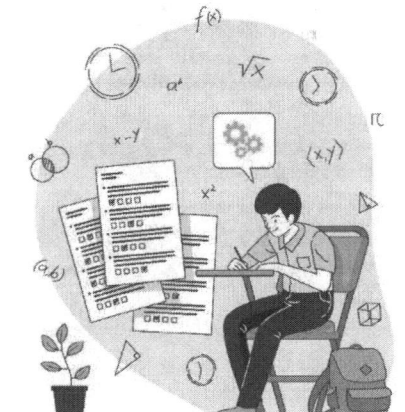

It's almost always better to start the guessing process too early than too late. It only takes a few seconds to remember something and answer the question from knowledge. Carefully eliminating wrong answer choices takes longer. Plus, going through the process of eliminating answer choices can actually help jog your memory.

**Summary**: Start the guessing process as soon as you decide that you can't answer the question based on your knowledge.

# How to Narrow Down the Choices

The next chapter in this book (**Test-Taking Strategies**) includes a wide range of strategies for how to approach questions and how to look for answer choices to eliminate. You will definitely want to read those carefully, practice them, and figure out which ones work best for you. Here though, we're going to address a mindset rather than a particular strategy.

Your odds of guessing an answer correctly depend on how many options you are choosing from.

| Number of options left | 5 | 4 | 3 | 2 | 1 |
|---|---|---|---|---|---|
| Odds of guessing correctly | 20% | 25% | 33% | 50% | 100% |

You can see from this chart just how valuable it is to be able to eliminate incorrect answers and make an educated guess, but there are two things that many test takers do that cause them to miss out on the benefits of guessing:

- Accidentally eliminating the correct answer
- Selecting an answer based on an impression

We'll look at the first one here, and the second one in the next section.

To avoid accidentally eliminating the correct answer, we recommend a thought exercise called **the $5 challenge**. In this challenge, you only eliminate an answer choice from contention if you are willing to bet $5 on it being wrong. Why $5? Five dollars is a small but not insignificant amount of money. It's an amount you could afford to lose but wouldn't want to throw away. And while losing

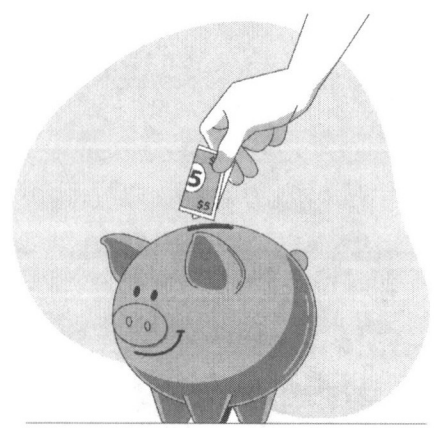

$5 once might not hurt too much, doing it twenty times will set you back $100. In the same way, each small decision you make—eliminating a choice here, guessing on a question there—won't by itself impact your score very much, but when you put them all together, they can make a big difference. By holding each answer choice elimination decision to a higher standard, you can reduce the risk of accidentally eliminating the correct answer.

The $5 challenge can also be applied in a positive sense: If you are willing to bet $5 that an answer choice *is* correct, go ahead and mark it as correct.

**Summary**: Only eliminate an answer choice if you are willing to bet $5 that it is wrong.

# Which Answer to Choose

You're taking the test. You've run into a hard question and decided you'll have to guess. You've eliminated all the answer choices you're willing to bet $5 on. Now you have to pick an answer. Why do we even need to talk about this? Why can't you just pick whichever one you feel like when the time comes?

The answer to these questions is that if you don't come into the test with a plan, you'll rely on your impression to select an answer choice, and if you do that, you risk falling into a trap. The test writers know that everyone who takes their test will be guessing on some of the questions, so they intentionally write wrong answer choices to seem plausible. You still have to pick an answer though, and if the wrong answer choices are designed to look right, how can you ever be sure that you're not falling for their trap? The best solution we've found to this dilemma is to take the decision out of your hands entirely. Here is the process we recommend:

**Once you've eliminated any choices that you are confident (willing to bet $5) are wrong, select the first remaining choice as your answer.**

Whether you choose to select the first remaining choice, the second, or the last, the important thing is that you use some preselected standard. Using this approach guarantees that you will not be enticed into selecting an answer choice that looks right, because you are not basing your decision on how the answer choices look.

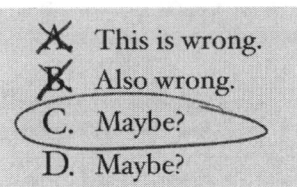

This is not meant to make you question your knowledge. Instead, it is to help you recognize the difference between your knowledge and your impressions. There's a huge difference between thinking an answer is right because of what you know, and thinking an answer is right because it looks or sounds like it should be right.

**Summary**: To ensure that your selection is appropriately random, make a predetermined selection from among all answer choices you have not eliminated.

# Test-Taking Strategies

This section contains a list of test-taking strategies that you may find helpful as you work through the test. By taking what you know and applying logical thought, you can maximize your chances of answering any question correctly!

It is very important to realize that every question is different and every person is different: no single strategy will work on every question, and no single strategy will work for every person. That's why we've included all of them here, so you can try them out and determine which ones work best for different types of questions and which ones work best for you.

## Question Strategies

### ✓ READ CAREFULLY

Read the question and the answer choices carefully. Don't miss the question because you misread the terms. You have plenty of time to read each question thoroughly and make sure you understand what is being asked. Yet a happy medium must be attained, so don't waste too much time. You must read carefully and efficiently.

### ✓ CONTEXTUAL CLUES

Look for contextual clues. If the question includes a word you are not familiar with, look at the immediate context for some indication of what the word might mean. Contextual clues can often give you all the information you need to decipher the meaning of an unfamiliar word. Even if you can't determine the meaning, you may be able to narrow down the possibilities enough to make a solid guess at the answer to the question.

### ✓ PREFIXES

If you're having trouble with a word in the question or answer choices, try dissecting it. Take advantage of every clue that the word might include. Prefixes can be a huge help. Usually, they allow you to determine a basic meaning. *Pre-* means before, *post-* means after, *pro-* is positive, *de-* is negative. From prefixes, you can get an idea of the general meaning of the word and try to put it into context.

### ✓ HEDGE WORDS

Watch out for critical hedge words, such as *likely, may, can, sometimes, often, almost, mostly, usually, generally, rarely,* and *sometimes*. Question writers insert these hedge phrases to cover every possibility. Often an answer choice will be wrong simply because it leaves no room for exception. Be on guard for answer choices that have definitive words such as *exactly* and *always*.

### ✓ SWITCHBACK WORDS

Stay alert for *switchbacks*. These are the words and phrases frequently used to alert you to shifts in thought. The most common switchback words are *but, although,* and *however*. Others include *nevertheless, on the other hand, even though, while, in spite of, despite,* and *regardless of*. Switchback words are important to catch because they can change the direction of the question or an answer choice.

## ⊘ FACE VALUE

When in doubt, use common sense. Accept the situation in the problem at face value. Don't read too much into it. These problems will not require you to make wild assumptions. If you have to go beyond creativity and warp time or space in order to have an answer choice fit the question, then you should move on and consider the other answer choices. These are normal problems rooted in reality. The applicable relationship or explanation may not be readily apparent, but it is there for you to figure out. Use your common sense to interpret anything that isn't clear.

# Answer Choice Strategies

## ⊘ ANSWER SELECTION

The most thorough way to pick an answer choice is to identify and eliminate wrong answers until only one is left, then confirm it is the correct answer. Sometimes an answer choice may immediately seem right, but be careful. The test writers will usually put more than one reasonable answer choice on each question, so take a second to read all of them and make sure that the other choices are not equally obvious. As long as you have time left, it is better to read every answer choice than to pick the first one that looks right without checking the others.

## ⊘ ANSWER CHOICE FAMILIES

An answer choice family consists of two (in rare cases, three) answer choices that are very similar in construction and cannot all be true at the same time. If you see two answer choices that are direct opposites or parallels, one of them is usually the correct answer. For instance, if one answer choice says that quantity *x* increases and another either says that quantity *x* decreases (opposite) or says that quantity *y* increases (parallel), then those answer choices would fall into the same family. An answer choice that doesn't match the construction of the answer choice family is more likely to be incorrect. Most questions will not have answer choice families, but when they do appear, you should be prepared to recognize them.

## ⊘ ELIMINATE ANSWERS

Eliminate answer choices as soon as you realize they are wrong, but make sure you consider all possibilities. If you are eliminating answer choices and realize that the last one you are left with is also wrong, don't panic. Start over and consider each choice again. There may be something you missed the first time that you will realize on the second pass.

## ⊘ AVOID FACT TRAPS

Don't be distracted by an answer choice that is factually true but doesn't answer the question. You are looking for the choice that answers the question. Stay focused on what the question is asking for so you don't accidentally pick an answer that is true but incorrect. Always go back to the question and make sure the answer choice you've selected actually answers the question and is not merely a true statement.

## ⊘ EXTREME STATEMENTS

In general, you should avoid answers that put forth extreme actions as standard practice or proclaim controversial ideas as established fact. An answer choice that states the "process should be used in certain situations, if..." is much more likely to be correct than one that states the "process should be discontinued completely." The first is a calm rational statement and doesn't even make a definitive, uncompromising stance, using a hedge word *if* to provide wiggle room, whereas the second choice is far more extreme.

### ⓧ Benchmark

As you read through the answer choices and you come across one that seems to answer the question well, mentally select that answer choice. This is not your final answer, but it's the one that will help you evaluate the other answer choices. The one that you selected is your benchmark or standard for judging each of the other answer choices. Every other answer choice must be compared to your benchmark. That choice is correct until proven otherwise by another answer choice beating it. If you find a better answer, then that one becomes your new benchmark. Once you've decided that no other choice answers the question as well as your benchmark, you have your final answer.

### ⓧ Predict the Answer

Before you even start looking at the answer choices, it is often best to try to predict the answer. When you come up with the answer on your own, it is easier to avoid distractions and traps because you will know exactly what to look for. The right answer choice is unlikely to be word-for-word what you came up with, but it should be a close match. Even if you are confident that you have the right answer, you should still take the time to read each option before moving on.

## General Strategies

### ⓧ Tough Questions

If you are stumped on a problem or it appears too hard or too difficult, don't waste time. Move on! Remember though, if you can quickly check for obviously incorrect answer choices, your chances of guessing correctly are greatly improved. Before you completely give up, at least try to knock out a couple of possible answers. Eliminate what you can and then guess at the remaining answer choices before moving on.

### ⓧ Check Your Work

Since you will probably not know every term listed and the answer to every question, it is important that you get credit for the ones that you do know. Don't miss any questions through careless mistakes. If at all possible, try to take a second to look back over your answer selection and make sure you've selected the correct answer choice and haven't made a costly careless mistake (such as marking an answer choice that you didn't mean to mark). This quick double check should more than pay for itself in caught mistakes for the time it costs.

### ⓧ Pace Yourself

It's easy to be overwhelmed when you're looking at a page full of questions; your mind is confused and full of random thoughts, and the clock is ticking down faster than you would like. Calm down and maintain the pace that you have set for yourself. Especially as you get down to the last few minutes of the test, don't let the small numbers on the clock make you panic. As long as you are on track by monitoring your pace, you are guaranteed to have time for each question.

### ⓧ Don't Rush

It is very easy to make errors when you are in a hurry. Maintaining a fast pace in answering questions is pointless if it makes you miss questions that you would have gotten right otherwise. Test writers like to include distracting information and wrong answers that seem right. Taking a little extra time to avoid careless mistakes can make all the difference in your test score. Find a pace that allows you to be confident in the answers that you select.

### ☑ Keep Moving

Panicking will not help you pass the test, so do your best to stay calm and keep moving. Taking deep breaths and going through the answer elimination steps you practiced can help to break through a stress barrier and keep your pace.

## Final Notes

The combination of a solid foundation of content knowledge and the confidence that comes from practicing your plan for applying that knowledge is the key to maximizing your performance on test day. As your foundation of content knowledge is built up and strengthened, you'll find that the strategies included in this chapter become more and more effective in helping you quickly sift through the distractions and traps of the test to isolate the correct answer.

Now that you're preparing to move forward into the test content chapters of this book, be sure to keep your goal in mind. As you read, think about how you will be able to apply this information on the test. If you've already seen sample questions for the test and you have an idea of the question format and style, try to come up with questions of your own that you can answer based on what you're reading. This will give you valuable practice applying your knowledge in the same ways you can expect to on test day.

**Good luck and good studying!**

# Clinical Classification Systems

## Interpreting Healthcare Data for Code Assignment

### COLLECTING ACCURATE HEALTHCARE DATA

Some benefits of capturing accurate healthcare data include:

- improving patients' quality of care
- identifying disparities in the delivery of health care
- enhancing healthcare research
- identifying disease trends that aid providers in resource management and cost effectiveness
- identifying opportunities to prevent fraudulent claims submission

Accurate data also assist healthcare management with fiscal planning, budgeting, development of initiatives to reduce patients' lengths of stay in the hospital, as well as unnecessary readmissions, and development of methods to prevent deaths. Associations such as Healthcare Information and Management Systems Society (HIMSS) aim to optimize health through clinical informatics or data analysis. Following suit, healthcare organizations have discovered the power of data when it comes to improving quality of care, and therefore, data accuracy is imperative to survival in the current healthcare realm.

### ROLE OF THE HIM EMPLOYEE

HIM professionals are essential team players in the capture of accurate healthcare data. A collaborative effort between HIM professionals and information technologists (IT) is key to the process of managing electronic information. HIM professionals may be involved in the process of managing electronic information through:

- data governance by establishing information management rules as a baseline
- data standardization through the creation and maintenance of a data dictionary
- data validation through the preservation of data integrity
- data analysis for the purpose of making informed decisions based upon reliable data

Additionally, HIM professionals are instrumental in the capture of accurate healthcare data for patient safety and quality improvement initiative. This process entails root-cause analysis of patient adverse events as well as the development of patient safety action plans. In terms of accurate data capture and its association with financial payment models, HIM professionals play an important role because of their ability to understand reimbursement methodologies.

### UNIFORM DATA COLLECTION PROCESS

Uniform Hospital Discharge Data Set (UHDDS) was established in 1974 by the US Department of Health and Human Services (HHS) for the purpose of establishing a minimum, common core data set. The data set is abstracted at the time of hospital discharge and the following elements are mandated for reporting: personal identification, date of birth, gender, race, ethnicity, residence, hospital identification, admission/discharge dates, type of admission, attending physician identification, operating physician identification, diagnoses, procedures with dates, patient disposition, and expected payer. Each of these UHDDS elements are captured on the insurance claims form known as the UB-04. Additionally, the UHDDS coincides with the requirements set forth by HIPAA, and is the standard followed by healthcare organizations to develop ICD coding/DRG reimbursement as well as statistical policies and procedures.

## DATA DICTIONARY

A data dictionary can be defined as a tool used by healthcare organizations for the purpose of ensuring accurate data collection. In order for data to be reliable and usable, all users and owners of the data must understand/interpret its meaning based upon the same source of truth—a data dictionary. According to a "Practice Brief" issued forth by the American Health Information Management Association (AHIMA), "standardizing data enhances interoperability across systems," and data dictionaries promote this necessary standardization. A data dictionary should describe the meaning of each data element. For example:

- naming conventions must match between systems
- definition of data elements must be explained
- field lengths of data elements should match between systems
- data types (e.g., alpha, numeric) should match between systems
- data frequency (e.g., monthly, annually) should match between systems

To reiterate, the primary goal of a data dictionary is to achieve standardization of data elements between various systems.

## ENSURING HEALTHCARE DATA ARE MEANINGFUL AND USEFUL

With healthcare initiatives focused upon quality, outcomes, and payment methodologies, it is a common practice for healthcare institutions to process their data so that they are meaningful; in other words, the purpose ultimately is to promote informed decision making. For data to be meaningful, they must first be captured, queried, and finally analyzed. Data capture should ensure that all the right information is collected and stored in an appropriate format. Data queries are conducted upon the collected information, but it is necessary for the data analyst to be familiar with all the systems where the data pulls from (e.g., EHR, pharmacy Pyxis systems, Chargemaster, computer-assisted coding [CAC], encoders). Data analysis should include quality checks, accurate interpretation through application of statistical formulas and/or algorithms, and presentation for informed decision making.

# Incorporating Clinical Vocabularies and Terminologies

## CLINICAL VOCABULARY

A clinical vocabulary (also known as clinical nomenclature) is best described as a list of clinical terms and their definitions/meanings. The clinical vocabulary list will be formally recognized by the healthcare entity as a list of *preferred* medical terms. The terms represent concepts, and the concepts can only have one meaning. In other words, the concepts are the foundation of the clinical vocabulary terms. The clinical vocabulary terms must: contain adequate content, be perpetual (meaning they are never deleted), be granular (detailed), be conceptually based (as discussed above), be understandable, and be useful. It is important to know that clinical vocabularies should be standardized so that ultimately, they promote data consistency, data quality, and enhance clinical work flows in the delivery of health care.

## MEDICAL CODING CLASSIFICATION SYSTEMS

A medical coding classification system is defined as a system that captures clinical data for reporting and reimbursement purposes. Reporting clinical data assists in statistical analyses of diseases as well as lending to decision support systems. There are two classification systems when it comes to medical coding that are widely recognized: International Classification of Diseases (ICD) and Current Procedural Terminology (CPT). The ICD system is an international classification system that identifies morbidity and mortality statistics. The version of ICD currently used in health care is the 10th version, also known as ICD-10. This version is divided into two components: ICD-10-CM (clinical modification) and ICD-10-PCS (procedure coding system). The CPT classification system was created for reporting purposes of care delivered by physicians. Other types of classification systems frequently referenced in healthcare billing and coding processes are Healthcare Common Procedure Coding Systems (HCPCS) as well as Diagnostic and Statistical Manual of Mental Disorders (DSM). Other entities that have alternate classification systems include home health, nursing, oncology, and pharmacotherapeutic.

## INTERNATIONAL CLASSIFICATION OF DISEASES

The development of the International Classification of Diseases (ICD) can be traced back to the 16th century where evidence exists of death records kept by London parishes. Substantial progress began to be made with classification systems, however, in 1893 when the Bertillon Classification of Diseases was developed. In 1900, the Bertillon Classification was renamed as the International Classification of Causes of Death, and has evolved over the years to the current International Classification of Diseases, 10th revision. Of interest, the 9th revision was used in the United States for 36 years (from 1979-2015). It consisted of 3 volumes, with the third volume designated for procedures. In preparing to transition to ICD-10, it became apparent that the original four-digit system was limited and needed substantial changes to accommodate technological advances in procedures. As a result, the International Classification of Diseases, 10th Revision, Procedure Coding System (ICD-10-PCS) was developed.

# Abstracting Information from Medical Records

## ABSTRACTING INFORMATION FROM MEDICAL RECORDS

Abstracting is the process of gleaning pertinent information from the medical record upon patient discharge. For healthcare entities still using paper records, data can be collected in two ways: either by manually completing a paper abstract or by manually keying in the information into a computerized database. More commonly in today's healthcare environment, automated abstracting is the common practice. Clinical abstracting software automates and streamlines the capture of pertinent data and is designed to easily analyze and generate reports of coded data, clinical data, research data, and reimbursement data. Efficient abstracting software aids in reducing billing delays. Encoders and computer-assisted coding (CAC) are instrumental in the automated abstracting process. CAC automatically mines for data through its natural language processor (NLP) tool, which is capable of identifying specific data from a patient's chart, and afterwards completes predefined templates designated by the healthcare entity.

## ABSTRACTING HEALTHCARE DATA

The primary reason to abstract healthcare data is to generate meaningful reports reflecting diagnoses encountered and treatment provided. As health care moves forward, "Big Data" becomes more relevant. Data provides a historical healthcare picture, the present-day situation, and predicts future performance models. The demands of regulatory agencies necessitate data abstraction and analysis. Meaningful use, population health, algorithms related to clinical informatics and reimbursement models, and healthcare reform are some examples of forces that push for data dependence and reliability. It is imperative that HIM professionals be subject matter experts of healthcare data abstraction and analysis. HIM professionals are the most knowledgeable when it comes to knowing how to gather meaningful data and how to manipulate it through EHR technology and reporting tools.

## HIM Professional's Role Pertaining to Data Integrity

The integrity of data in a healthcare organization should not be solely the responsibility of Information Technology (IT). HIM should be an integral member of the healthcare organization's data governance team. HIM should play a leading role in the development and implementation of data integrity best practices. HIM professionals are those individuals who are trained to identify data discrepancies, such as duplicate records. HIM can analyze algorithms and their associated data fields, and subsequently detect incorrect or inaccurate record matching. It also is imperative that HIM and IT collaborate during data mapping processes, again aiming to correctly map data fields and test the work flow to ensure errors are identified prior to implementation.

# Consulting Reference Materials

## Official Sources of Truth When Assigning ICD-10 Codes

With the implementation of ICD-10 in October 2015, dependence upon reference materials for proper coding guidance are more important than ever to a medical coder. To compound the new codes, new technologies also add a layer of complexity (e.g., CAC and NLP), not to mention hybrid record systems (paper and EHRs). Of course, logic-based encoders and advanced electronic coding references are helpful in making decisions regarding correct coding practices. Some of the most common coding references widely used are: American Hospital Association's (AHA) Coding Clinic for ICD-9 and ICD-10; American Medical Association's (AMA) CPT Assistant; National Correct Coding Initiatives (NCCI); CPT Changes: An Insider's View; Coder's Desk Reference (CDR); Medical Acronyms & Abbreviations List; Disease Process Manuals; and Drug Reference tools. Additionally, HIM-related associations (AHIMA and AAPC) offer other reliable resources (e.g., newsletters, forums, publications, online coding help). Final coding disagreements can be resolved by consulting coding professionals through a paid subscription to 3M Nosology.

## Supporting Assigned Codes with Reliable Reference Sources

The use of reliable reference sources in support of code assignments is an absolute necessity as a coder. Inevitably, denials of submitted claims will be received by a healthcare organization. In order to appeal a denial (e.g., RAC) and ultimately win the appeal, supportive documentation is key. Through the utilization of reliable resources, arguments by third party payers against codes assigned by the healthcare organization are invalid. It is always pertinent for a coder and/or internal coding auditor to reference these sources of truth so that overcoding, upcoding, and/or unbundling of codes are avoided, and subsequent external audits are potentially avoided as well. Furthermore, reliable reference sources can provide guidance to aid in avoiding false claims submission as well as ensure compliance with external regulatory agencies (e.g., OIG, RAC, CMS).

## Browsing the Internet for References Applicable to Coding Situations

Some of the most common coding references used by coders are available through an encoder or a computer-assisted coding (CAC) software program. However, there are times when these references do not address the current coding scenario. For example, a complicated operation (e.g., spinal fusion) utilizing various devices (e.g., cages, implants, stimulators, bone graft) from multiple suppliers (e.g., Arthrex, DePuy, Medtronic, Siemens) can be overwhelming to a coder. It is appropriate for the coder to browse the Internet for articles or videos that describe or show the actual procedure in progress. These educational venues enable the coder to better understand the procedure and subsequently be able to choose the appropriate code(s).

# Applying Coding Guidelines

## INPATIENT

### FOLLOWING INPATIENT CODING GUIDELINES

The ICD-10-CM and ICD-10-PCS official guidelines for coding and reporting are provided by the Centers for Medicare and Medicaid Services (CMS) and the National Center for Health Statistics (NCHS) primarily as companion documents to the ICD-10 coding books. The coding guidelines are a set of rules that correspond to the coding conventions and instructions. Adherence to these guidelines is mandated by the Health Information Portability and Accountability Act (HIPAA). The guidelines are a source of truth when it comes to answering difficult coding questions. They are a central reference place for coders, managers, and auditors (internal and external) to access when reaching a compromise in difficult coding scenarios. They promote consistency among coders and healthcare providers in the assignment of codes.

> **Review Video: HIPAA**
> Visit mometrix.com/academy and enter code: 412009

### APPLYING CODING CONVENTIONS WHEN ASSIGNING CODES

Correct assignment of ICD-10-CM/PCS codes is contingent upon each coder's comprehension of the coding conventions. With the use of computer-assisted coding and/or encoders as well as just having the basic knowledge of the conventions, most coders do not really think about the coding conventions. However, a thorough understanding of their meanings and purpose is essential to the correct assignment of codes. The conventions each have a special meaning in ICD-10, such as follows:

| Convention | Meaning/Purpose |
|---|---|
| Placeholder Character | The letter "X" is used to provide future expansion of a code. |
| Seventh Characters | Some codes need a 7th character for provide further specificity |
| Abbreviations | Not Elsewhere Classified (NEC) and Not Otherwise Specified (NOS) |
| Punctuation | Parentheses are used to enclose supplementary words; brackets are used to synonyms and/or manifestation codes; colons are used to indicate an incomplete term that needs additional information. |
| Instructional Notes | Includes/Excludes notes, "Code First" notes, "Use Additional Code," etc. |
| Relational Terms | "And" means "and/or," and "With" means "associated with" or "due to" |

### HIERARCHICAL STRUCTURE OF ICD-10-CM

The hierarchical structure of ICD-**10**-CM is similar to ICD-**9**-CM in that the first three characters of the codes are categorized according to similar traits. The differences between the two editions are below:

| Differences | ICD-10 | ICD-9 |
|---|---|---|
| Number of Chapters | 21 | 17 |
| Code Structure | Alphanumeric, Length = 3 to 7 characters | Numeric, Length = 3 to 5 characters |

| Differences | ICD-10 | ICD-9 |
|---|---|---|
| Diseases of the Sensory Organs | Eyes/Ears separated into own chapter | Combined in the Nervous System Diseases |
| Injury Classification | According to site (e.g., arm) | According to type (e.g., wound) |
| Placeholder | "X" is used when a code has less than 6 characters but a 7th character is required. | None |
| V & E supplemental codes | Incorporated into main classification system | Available for assignment |
| Titles | Includes full titles for codes | Refers the coder back to common 4th and 5th digits |

These ICD-10-CM changes are a significant improvement from the 9th edition.

## New Features of ICD-10-CM in Comparison to ICD-9-CM

There are numerous new features of ICD-**10**-CM in comparison to ICD-**9**-CM, all aimed at providing a greater level of specificity and clinical detail. The new features are updated to be more consistent with modern clinical practices. The new features are as follows:

- New combination codes
- Added laterality
- Added 7th character for episode of care
- Expanded codes
- Inclusion of trimesters in obstetrical codes
- Changes in time frames for acute myocardial infarctions (8 weeks decreased to 4 weeks) and abortions versus fetal death (22 weeks decreased to 20 weeks)
- Changes in definitions of exclusion notes (e.g., Excludes1 and Excludes2)

These new features will provide data that enhances quality of care, enhances reimbursement models, improves research and clinical trial studies, and enhances the monitoring of resource usage

## Coding Specificity from Ancillary Reports for Inpatient Accounts

Ancillary services typically refer to diagnostic services that originate in radiology and pathology. These services are provided by radiologists and pathologists, who are physicians. Therefore, it would seem that it would be appropriate to code their services. However, coding guidelines instruct coders to *not* assign codes based on x-ray results or pathology reports for inpatient accounts unless the treating physician documents their clinical significance. This guidance is based on the fact that these diagnostic results are open to interpretation and must be validated by the treating physician through his/her medical decision-making process. The decision must be documented separately from the ancillary report, and at that point, the coder may consider this documentation for coding purposes. Additionally, laboratory services are also ancillary, and their results require a treating physician's interpretation and documentation before coding.

## Attributes of ICD-10-PCS Codes

The structure of ICD-9, Volume 3, for procedural coding was not capable of evolving into more codes necessary for keeping up with the explosion of technological advances in health care. Therefore, it became mandatory in the ICD-10 realm for procedure codes to be designed in such a way as to accommodate growth long-term. The result was ICD-10-PCS (Procedural Coding System) with elimination of a third volume (as was used in ICD-9). ICD-10-PCS was developed with four major attributes and their meanings in mind: completeness (one unique code for each different procedure), expandability (ICD-10-PCS allows for the incorporation of new procedure codes), multiaxial (codes consist of independent characters with the capability to retain meaning across broad ranges of codes), and standardized terminology (each term must have a specific meaning). It is important that coders thoroughly understand the definitions for all the procedures and the various approaches to operations as this will be key to correct code assignments.

## GENERAL PRINCIPLES TO FOLLOW WHEN DEVELOPING ICD-10-PCS CODES

The structure of ICD-9, Volume 3, for procedural coding was not capable of evolving into more codes necessary for keeping up with the explosion of technological advances in healthcare. Therefore, it became mandatory in the ICD-10 realm for procedure codes to be designed in such a way as to accommodate growth long-term. The result was ICD-10-PCS (Procedural Coding System) with elimination of a third volume (as was used in ICD-9). ICD-10-PCS was developed following several general principles: 1) diagnostic information is no longer included in the procedural codes; 2) there is less usage of the not otherwise specified (NOS) designation; 3) there is limited usage of the not elsewhere classified (NEC) designation; and, 4) there is expansion of the level of specificity.

## ICD-10-PCS FORMAT

ICD-10-PCS is formatted in three sections: Tables, Index, and List of Codes. The Index is an alphabetic listing of procedures/operations. Codes are organized in the Index according to the general type of procedure. Of note, the Index only provides the first 3 to 4 characters of a procedural code. The remaining characters are located in the tables, and thus the tables must be referenced in order to assign a valid 7-digit code. The tables are designed in rows that provide options for characters 4 to 7 in the development of valid code combinations. The List of Codes is a comprehensive list of all procedural codes along with their descriptions. The process of assigning an ICD-10-PCS code begins with the coder accessing the Index in order to locate the appropriate table, and then referencing that table to locate the remaining characters for code completion.

## CHARACTERS FOR MEDICAL AND SURGICAL PROCEDURES

Medical and surgical procedural codes are composed of 7 characters. The characters and their meaning follow. The first character represents 4 different *sections*: 0 – Med/Surg; 1 – Obstetrics; 2 – Placement; and, 3 – Administration. (The majority of procedural codes are categorized in the Med/Surg section.) The second character represents the *body system* (e.g., cardiology, respiratory). The third character represents the *root operation*, also known as the objective of the procedure. The fourth character represents the *body part* where the procedure is performed (e.g., stomach, brain). The fifth character represents the *approach* or method to reach the procedure site (e.g., open, percutaneous). The sixth character represents the *device* used during the procedure (e.g., implant). The seventh character represents the *qualifier* that provides additional information about the procedure. Tip to memorizing the 7 characters:

| Section | Sam |
|---|---|
| Body System | Baked |
| Root Operation | Raspberry |
| Body Part | Bagels |
| Approach | And |
| Device | Delicious |
| Qualifier | Quiche |

## Root Operations Wherein the Objective Is to Pull Out/Off All or a Portion of a Body Part

There are five root operations in ICD-10-PCS that remove some or all of a body part. All five are done with no replacement of the body part or tissue. The five root operations are listed as follows (with their differences in bold):

| Root Operation | Purpose of the Procedure | Site of Procedure |
| --- | --- | --- |
| Excision | Cut out or off | Portion of a body part |
| Resection | Cut out or off | Entire body part |
| Detachment | Cut out or off | Extremities only; exclusive to amputations |
| Destruction | Eradicate/Destroy | Body part not removed, rather destroyed |
| Extraction | Pull out with force | Portion of a body part or entire body part |

Of note, there are 31 root operations in total, divided into 9 groups that are similar. The remaining eight groups are procedures that: 1) remove solids/fluids/gases, 2) cut or separate only, 3) put in or put back some or all of a body part, 4) alter the diameter of a tubular structure, 5) include a device, 6) involve examination only, 7) include other repairs, and, 8) include other objectives.

## Root Operations That Always Involve a Device

Six root operations in ICD-10-PCS always involve a device. For the purposes of ICD-10-PCS coding, a device is defined as an appliance or material that remains in the body or on the body after the procedure. The six root operations are listed as follows (with their differences in bold):

| Root Operation | Purpose of the Procedure | Example |
| --- | --- | --- |
| Insertion | Addition of a non-biological device | Foley catheter placement |
| Replacement | Addition of a device that replaces a body part | Phacoemulsification with IOL implant |
| Supplement | Addition of a device that reinforces a body part | Umbilical hernia repair with mesh |
| Change | Exchange of a device | Tracheostomy tube exchange |
| Removal | Take out a device | Removal of endotracheal tube |
| Revision | Modification of a malfunctioning device | Adjustment of a pacemaker lead |

## Assignment of a POA Indicator for a Combination Code That Identifies Both the Chronic Condition and the Acute Exacerbation

Present on Admission (POA) indicators are a reporting requirement for healthcare providers. The Deficit Reduction Act of 2005 mandated that providers report whether diseases were present on admission or not. The intent of the indicators is to differentiate between conditions that are present at the time of admission and those that develop during the inpatient admission. Financial incentives are available for providers who reduce the number of hospital-acquired conditions (not present on admission). There are five indicators to select from: "Y" = yes, POA; "N" = no, not POA; "U" = unknown, documentation is insufficient to make a determination; "W" = clinically undetermined; and, "1" = exempt from POA reporting. In the instance where a combination code identifies both a chronic condition as well as its acute exacerbation, the following best practice should be followed: Assign "N" if any part of the combination code was not POA; assign "Y" if all parts of the combination code were POA.

## Determining "Upper" and "Lower" Body Parts in ICD-10-PCS Coding

In ICD-10-PCS coding, in some scenarios, a coder will encounter documentation referring to "upper" or "lower" body parts. For example, the documentation may refer to upper or lower arteries or veins. When the terms "upper" or "lower" are used in reference to body parts, the dividing anatomical line between the two body locations is the diaphragm. Understanding this general guideline will aid the coder in selecting the correct body system that represents character #2 of the procedural code.

## Determine ICD-10-PCS Coding If an Intended Procedure Is Discontinued

In some instances, an operative procedure is discontinued for various reasons. When this occurs, the coder must determine to what extent the procedure was conducted. Once this is determined, the coder should code the procedure to the appropriate root operation. For example, a laparoscopic cholecystectomy is planned, and the laparoscope is inserted into the abdominal cavity, but the patient becomes hypotensive and the surgery is stopped. In this case, the coder would code the laparoscopic approach only. In other instances, a root operation may not even be performed. In that case, a code should be assigned for inspection of the appropriate body part. Understanding this general guideline will aid the coder in selecting the correct root operation that represents character #3 of the procedural code.

## Determining the Appropriate Code Assignment When a Biopsy Is Followed by More Definitive Treatment

When a biopsy of a site leads to more definitive treatment (such as excision of the diseased site), both the biopsy and the more definitive treatment are coded. A good example of this guideline is when a biopsy of the breast is positive for carcinoma, and the physician decides to proceed with a lumpectomy, partial mastectomy, or even a total mastectomy during the same operative episode. The act of proceeding with a more definitive procedure is a common practice. This guideline differs from ICD-9 procedural coding.

# Outpatient

## Following Outpatient Coding Guidelines

The Current Procedural Terminology (CPT) code set is the most widely accepted nomenclature for the reporting of physician procedures and services. It is endorsed by the HHS as the nationally accepted coding standard. Each section of the CPT code book includes specific guidelines. These coding guidelines are a set of rules for coders to follow in order to appropriately interpret and report procedures and services provided in physician's offices and/or outpatient settings. As with all coding guidelines, they promote consistency amongst coders and healthcare providers in the assignment of codes.

## Current Procedural Terminology Book

The Current Procedural Terminology (CPT) book was originally published in 1966. It is used to assign codes for procedures and/or services provided by a physician in his/her office, or provided in an outpatient setting such as a surgery center. The CPT book is published by the American Medical Association (AMA) and is updated annually by a CPT editorial panel and advisory committee comprised of healthcare professionals. The CPT procedural codes are used alongside ICD-10-CM diagnostic codes on claims, and both sets of codes are analyzed by payers for reimbursement purposes. The CPT book is composed of an introduction section (instructions for using the book), six main sections (e.g., evaluation and management, anesthesia, surgery, radiology, pathology/laboratory, and medicine), 13 appendices (e.g., modifiers, summary of add-on codes, clinical examples, etc.), Category II and III codes (supplemental and/or temporary codes), and an alphabetic index.

## Coding Guideline for Assignment of the First-Listed Condition (Diagnosis) for Outpatient Stays

When assigning diagnostic codes for an outpatient encounter, a "principal diagnosis" would not be assigned for outpatient services because principal diagnosis refers solely to an inpatient admission. Rather, for outpatient services, the reason for the encounter or visit is called the first-listed diagnosis (also referred to as the primary diagnosis). The first-listed or primary diagnosis is determined based upon the patient's presentation to the hospital. For example, when a patient presents for outpatient surgery, the coder would select the reason for the surgery as the first-listed diagnosis. This would be the case even if the surgery was canceled for any reason. In another scenario, when a patient is admitted to the hospital as an observation patient for a medical condition, the coder would select the reason for the medical condition as the first-listed diagnosis. There are times when a patient develops complications from an outpatient surgical procedure and is subsequently admitted to the hospital under observation status. In those instances, the coder would assign the primary diagnosis as the reason for the surgery followed by codes for the complications that necessitated the admission to observation status.

## Services Included in a CPT Surgical Code

There are certain services that are always bundled into the CPT surgical code in addition to the actual operation. Since the services are bundled into one CPT surgical code, they are not "unbundled," meaning they are not coded separately. The following services are included in the CPT code:

- local infiltration, anesthetic block, or topical anesthesia
- one evaluation and management (E/M) encounter on the date immediately prior to the procedure or on the date of the procedure
- immediate postoperative care
- physician orders
- evaluation of the patient in the postanesthesia recovery area
- typical postoperative follow-up care

This bundled group of services is also referred to as a CPT Surgical Package.

## Modifiers

Modifiers are used quite frequently with CPT codes. Their purpose is to indicate that the procedure has been altered in some way from the usual procedural process. With the application of modifiers, the assignment of extra separate procedure codes is avoided. Some examples of when modifiers may be used are for:

- a service or procedure performed by more than one physician and/or in more than one location
- a service or procedure increased (e.g., work required to complete the procedure is extensively greater than expected) or reduced (e.g., procedure partially completed or canceled)
- a procedure required a significant and separately identifiable E/M service by the same physician on the same day as the procedure
- a procedure was performed on bilateral locations (e.g., both extremities)
- a service or procedure was provided more than once

## RELEVANCE OF TIME TO CPT CODE SELECTION

Time is an important factor when considering the assignment of some CPT codes. Time is understood to be the amount of time when the healthcare provider is face-to-face with the patient (e.g., evaluation and management services). It is also important to understand the definition of a "unit of time." A unit of time is based on when the midpoint is passed (e.g., 31 minutes would be past the midpoint of 0 to 60 minutes). Correct time calculations in the assignment of codes for drug or hydration infusions can be challenging secondary to numerous instructions, hierarchical rules, and different payer policies. Beyond these challenges, time factors vary depending on the method of drug administration (injection, infusion, or a push). For example, a drug "injection" typically takes about 3 to 5 minutes to perform, whereas a drug "infusion" usually lasts for 30 minutes or more. An IV "push" is an infusion of 15 minutes or less. Therefore, an initial "infusion" will be at least 16 minutes and could last up to 90 minutes. Additional hours of infusion are calculated in increments of 30 minutes. These three types of drug administration examples provide a clear picture of the relevance of time with CPT code selection.

## CODE SYMBOLS USED IN THE CPT CODEBOOK

Code symbols are used in the CPT code book to facilitate quick understanding. They primarily represent additions, deletions, and revisions. A quick reference table of the symbols and their meanings are noted here:

| Symbol | | Meaning |
|---|---|---|
| Bullet | ● | New procedure code |
| Triangle | ▲ | Revised procedure code |
| Facing triangles | ►◄ | New and revised information in the CPT guidelines |
| Plus sign | + | Add-on code |
| Circle | ○ | Code has been reinstated |
| Circled bullet | ◉ | Use of moderate sedation |
| Null zero | ⊘ | CPT codes that may not be used with modifier -51 |
| Flash symbol | ⚡ | Products pending FDA approval |

## PHYSICIAN

### EVALUATION AND MANAGEMENT SECTION OF THE CPT CODE BOOK

The evaluation and management (E/M) section of the CPT code book is divided into general categories of office visits, hospital visits, and consultations. These categories are further subdivided into subcategories. For example, the office visit category has subcategories pertaining to new patients and established patients. Hospital visits have subcategories pertaining to initial and subsequent visits. Formatting similarities between the different categories are: unique codes are listed first, followed by the place and/or type of service (e.g., outpatient visit), followed by the content of the service noted (e.g., problem-focused physical exam), followed by the nature of the problem (e.g., the patient has developed a significant complication), and concluded with a time element associated with the service/procedure (e.g., 15 minutes at the bedside).

### DEFINITIONS OF NEW AND ESTABLISHED PATIENTS WHEN ASSIGNING E/M CODES

In order to assign the correct evaluation and management (E/M) code, it is necessary to understand the difference between a new patient and an established patient. The difference is easy to understand because essentially it is based on a time frame of 3 years. In other words, if a patient has received professional services (e.g., face-to-face time with a physician or even services from a physician of the exact same specialty belonging to the same group practice) within the last 3 years, then he/she is considered to be an established patient. If the patient has not received the professional services within the past 3 years (e.g., same physician practice conditions), then he/she is considered to be a new patient. These principles do not apply for a patient being seen in an emergency department.

## COMPONENTS FOR THE LEVELS OF E/M SERVICES

For a coder to determine an appropriate evaluation and management (E/M) code, he/she must review documentation to identify the seven components that define the various levels of E/M services. The components to consider are history, examination, medical decision making, counseling, coordination of care, nature of presenting problem, and time. History, examination, and medical decision making are known to be the key components in selecting an E/M level. The following three components are known as contributory factors: The history refers to the chief complaint, the history of present illness, etc. The examination refers to the extent of the physical exam. Medical decision making refers to the complexity of establishing a diagnosis. Counseling refers to a discussion between the physician and the patient. The nature of the presenting problem can refer to a disease, condition, injury, symptom, etc. Time is included as a component to aid the physician in selecting the most appropriate level of E/M service.

## TYPES OF PRESENTING PROBLEMS FOR E/M CODING

When assigning an evaluation and management (E/M) code, a coder must determine the type of presenting problem the patient has acquired. The presenting problem could be an illness, an injury, a sign or symptom, etc., and there may not even be a diagnosis determined by the physician at the time of the patient's presentation. The E/M codes recognize five types of presenting problems. They are minimal, minor, low severity, moderate severity, and high severity. An example of a minimal problem would be one that does not require the presence of a physician, but the service is provided under the physician's supervision. A minor problem would be one that passes quickly and does not likely affect the patient's health status permanently. A low-severity problem is one wherein the risk associated with the illness/injury with no treatment is low, and a full recovery is expected. A moderate severity problem is recognized as one wherein the risk associated with the illness/injury without treatment is moderate and a risk of death is moderate as well. A high-severity problem is one in which the risk of the illness/injury without treatment is high, and there is probable severe impairment to the patient's health status.

## SELECTING A LEVEL OF E/M SERVICE

There are instructions for a coder to follow when selecting the appropriate level of evaluation and management (E/M) service. The first step is to review the reporting instructions that are unique to the selected category or subcategory. Next, review the level of E/M service descriptors in the selected category/subcategory. These descriptors refer to the components of E/M levels: history, examination, medical decision making, counseling, coordination of care, nature of presenting problem, and time. In terms of the history, the coder must determine the extent of history obtained (e.g., problem focused, expanded problem focused, detailed, or comprehensive). In terms of the extent of the examination performed, the coder must determine if it is problem focused, expanded problem focused, detailed, or comprehensive. Determining the complexity of the medical decision making entails whether it was straightforward, low complexity, moderate complexity, or high complexity. Time is a significant factor to determine as well because it will aid the physician in selecting the appropriate level of service.

# Assigning Codes

## INPATIENT CODES

### CODE STRUCTURE OF AN ICD-10-CM CODE

Unlike ICD-**9**-CM code assignments that only contained 3 to 5 characters, ICD-**10**-CM codes contain anywhere from 3 to 7 characters. The first character of the ICD-10-CM code will always be one of the following alphabetic letters: A-T and V-Z. Note, the letter "U" is not used because it has been reserved by the World Health Organization (WHO) for other purposes. The second character of the ICD-10-CM code will always be numeric, and the remaining characters can be either alpha or numeric. The decimal is still used after the third character in the ICD-**10**-CM code just as it was in the ICD-**9**-CM code. Secondary to the expansion of the code structure to up to 7 characters, there are now more than 68,000 codes, compared with only 13,000 codes in ICD-9. The expansion of the code structure allows for greater specificity and clinical detail.

### ICD-10-CM TABULAR LIST

The key to understanding the ICD-10-CM tabular list is to be aware of how it is categorized and subcategorized. The first principle to understand is that the list is divided into 21 chapters. The following table depicts part of the breakdown of chapter 1 as an example:

| Chapter | Block | Sub-Category |
|---|---|---|
| Chapter 1 - Certain infectious and parasitic diseases (A00-B99) | A00-A09 Intestinal infectious diseases | A00.0 Cholera due to *Vibrio cholerae* 01, biovar cholerae: Classical cholera |
| | | A00.1 Cholera due to *Vibrio cholerae* 01, biovar eltor: Cholera eltor |
| | | A00.9 Cholera, unspecified |
| | | A01.0 Typhoid fever: Infection due to *Salmonella typhi* |
| | | ⋮ |
| | A15-A19 Tuberculosis | A15.0 Tuberculosis of lung |
| | | A15.4 Tuberculosis of intrathoracic lymph nodes |
| | | ⋮ |

A coder must process through each available category in order to assign the code with the highest level of specificity, which for some codes will only be 3 characters, and for other codes, 7 characters. For those codes with a 7th character that explains whether it is an initial or subsequent encounter or the sequelae of a previous disease/condition, it may be necessary to use the placeholder character of "X" to fill in for any empty spaces.

## ICD-10-CM ALPHABETIC INDEX

The ICD-10-CM alphabetic index is similarly arranged to the ICD-9-CM alphabetic index with a few differences. The following table demonstrates their similarities and differences:

| CD Version | Index to Diseases & Injuries | Index to External Causes | Hypertension Table | Table of Drugs & Chemicals |
|---|---|---|---|---|
| ICD-9-CM | Yes | Yes | Yes | Yes |
| ICD-10-CM | Yes | Yes | No | Yes |

Main terms in the ICD-10-CM alphabetic index are in bold font and vertically aligned with the left-hand margin. Indented beneath each main term are subterms with the corresponding code to be further researched in the tabular list. Only the first 4 characters of the code are listed. If additional characters are required, a dash (-) will be present at the end of the index entry. Morphology codes are no longer included in the alphabetic index for ICD-10-CM, but manifestation codes are still included in the same manner as ICD-9-CM.

In the ICD-10-CM code book, there are two abbreviations used as conventions that affect code assignment. They are: Not Elsewhere Classified (NEC) and Not Otherwise Specified (NOS). The purpose behind their use is identical to ICD-9-CM coding; however, they are not used as frequently in ICD-10-CM. Not Elsewhere Classified means when a specific code is not available for a condition, then this "other specified" code is selected for code assignment. Not Otherwise Specified means the physician has not provided sufficient documentation to support assignment of a more specific code. It is important to remember that the NOS abbreviation is *not* used in ICD-10-PCS procedural coding. This is because ICD-10-PCS requires a minimal level of specificity in order to construct a code. NOS is used in ICD-10-PCS coding, but its use is limited.

## PUNCTUATION MARKS USED IN ICD-10-CM CODING

The following punctuation marks are used throughout the ICD-10-CM code book: parentheses, brackets, and colons. They are used in both the Alphabetic Index as well as the Tabular List. Parentheses are used to enclose supplementary words associated with a disease. These words are referred to as *nonessential* modifiers because the presence or absence of these terms has no effect on the selection of the code. (Of note, subterms that have their own line entry below the main term are referred to as *essential* modifiers, and they do have an effect on code selection.) Brackets are used to enclose synonyms or further explanation of terms. They are also used to indicate manifestation codes in the Alphabetic Index. Colons are used to indicate an incomplete term that needs an additional modifier indented under the main term in order to assign the correct code.

## PURPOSE BEHIND INSTRUCTIONAL NOTES IN THE ALPHABETIC INDEX AND TABULAR LIST OF ICD-10-CM

Instructional notes are still used in the ICD-10 books. The different types of notes are: inclusion notes, exclusion notes, code first notes, use additional code notes, and cross-reference notes (e.g., *see, see also,* and *see condition*). The inclusion notes are easy to identify because they are introduced with the word "includes" at the beginning of a category, chapter, or section. Exclusion notes are divided into two types: *Excludes1* or *Excludes2*. *Excludes1* means that a code is "not coded here" or that the code should never be used simultaneously as the code above the *Excludes1* note. *Excludes2* means that "not included here." In other words, the excluded condition is not part of the condition represented by the code, and, therefore, the two codes can be coded together if the patient has been diagnosed with both conditions. Code first and use additional code notes are similar to ICD-9 guidelines and represent underlying conditions along with their manifestations. Cross-reference notes instruct the coder to look elsewhere before assigning a code.

## PROCESS OF USING THE ICD-10-PCS INDEX TO LOCATE A PROCEDURE

A coder should first reference the ICD-10-PCS index to begin the process of locating the most appropriate code for the procedure performed. The procedural codes are organized in the index based upon the general type of procedure (e.g., excision, dilation, repair, removal). The index outlines the first three or four characters of a code, which the coder uses to reference the corresponding ICD-10-PCS table for the purpose of completing the code. The coder must reference the table in order to obtain a complete and valid procedural code. The principle of referencing the ICD-10-PCS table is similar to the principle in ICD-9 coding when the coder was expected to reference the tabular list to obtain a valid code.

## LAYOUT OF THE ICD-10-PCS TABLE

A coder must use the ICD-10-PCS table to obtain complete and valid procedural codes. The table is constructed with a top and bottom portion. The top portion of the table reflects the first three characters of the code (already determined from the ICD-10-PCS index). The bottom portion of the table reflects all valid combinations of code characters four through seven. The fourth through seventh characters must be selected from the same row of data as it expands across the four columns pertaining to the body part, procedural approach, device, and qualifier. It is important to understand that characters four through seven cannot be selected just anywhere on the table; rather, the selections must remain within the same row. The options for code selections per table are innumerable.

## OUTPATIENT CODES

### SELECTING A CPT CODE FROM THE CPT INDEX

In order to select an appropriate CPT procedural code form the CPT code book, the coder should access the index found the back of the code book. The alphabetic index is organized according to four categories of main entries. The main entries can be located by:

- procedure or service name
- organ or anatomical site
- condition
- synonyms/ eponyms/abbreviations

After locating the appropriate main terms in the index, a coder may also notice modifying terms or subterms. These modifying terms/subterms are words that further expound upon the main term. It is important to remember that the index should only be the beginning of the search for an appropriate code. The coder must continue on with the process by researching the main text of the CPT code book to ensure the correct code has been selected.

### SERVICES INCLUDED IN ANESTHESIA CPT CODES

CPT codes not only exist for procedural codes, but they also are available for anesthesia services. The code range for these codes is 00100-01999. Anesthesia services are provided by an anesthesiologist or by a certified registered nurse anesthetist under the supervision of an anesthesiologist. The anesthesia codes can include the services of general, regional, or local anesthesia, preoperative and postoperative visits by the anesthesiologist, anesthetic care during the procedure, monitoring of vital signs, and administration of blood, fluid, or drugs. When attempting to locate an applicable anesthetic code, the coder should realize that the codes are organized in the code book by anatomic site. There is also a set of anesthesia physical status modifiers (P1 through

P6), which may be assigned in addition to the anesthesia CPT code for the purpose of indicating the patient's overall health status (e.g., healthy patient, mild systemic disease).

## SURGERY SECTION IN THE CPT BOOK

The CPT Surgery section of the CPT book is organized according to body systems (e.g., General, Cardiovascular system, Respiratory system, Nervous system). Each of the surgical categories is further subdivided according to organs, anatomical sites, and types of procedures. In order to locate procedures in the Surgery section, the coder will first need to reference the CPT alphabetic index, searching for either the name of the procedure, the type of procedure, or anatomical site. In the index, the coder will notice a range of codes, for which he/she will reference in the main text of the code book, and then subsequently select the most appropriate CPT code within that range.

## CMS'S GLOBAL SURGERY CONCEPT

CMS has defined the global surgery concept (also known as a surgical package) as a range of services included in an operation. From a reimbursement perspective, the surgical package is understood to be bundled under the appropriate corresponding CPT procedural code. The bundled package includes the following: administration of anesthetic products, one related evaluation and management (E/M) service on the day of or the day prior to the surgery, immediate postoperative care, physician orders, postanesthesia care in the recovery room, and standard postoperative care follow-up. A coder should never unbundle the surgical package and bill the components separately as this would constitute fraud. It is also important to remember that other third-party payers aside from Medicare may define the surgical package differently.

## PROFESSIONAL COMPONENT VS. TECHNICAL COMPONENT OF A CPT CODE

The differences between the professional component of a service and the technical component of the same service can be a confusing topic for coders to understand. As a result, sometimes healthcare entities will establish their charges for technical services based solely on professional service documentation, which is an incorrect practice. The professional component includes the physician's supervision of the service, reading, and interpreting test results, and documentation of the report's interpretation. On the other hand, the technical component of a service is the use of equipment, facilities, non-physician staff, and supplies to perform the service. Technical charges will never include the physician's professional fees. An easy way to remember the technical component is to think of it as the healthcare entity's overhead. For example, a patient undergoes an MRI. On the claim, the applicable MRI charge would be included with the "TC" modifier (to indicate the technical component) as the healthcare entity would be seeking reimbursement for the use of the MRI equipment, the cost of any contrast used (supplies), and the cost of the MRI technician's time used to operate the MRI equipment.

## PHYSICIAN CODES

### ENCOUNTER FORM/SUPERBILL

An encounter form can also be referred to as a superbill, charge slip, or routing form. It is a source document that collects information pertaining to the patient's diagnostic and treatment information as well as financial information. These preprinted forms are used in a physician's office/clinic, and are composed of the following sections: an examination and treatment section of typical evaluation and management (E/M) codes and/or CPT codes, diagnosis codes, comments, and demographic/billing information. The physician or healthcare provider is responsible for completing the form based on their clinical judgment, and the billing clerk enters the selected charges onto the claim form.

## IF IT ISN'T DOCUMENTED, IT HASN'T BEEN DONE

The statement, "If it isn't documented, it hasn't been done," has been a long-standing adage well known to health information professionals. Healthcare provider documentation of diagnoses and treatment rendered is the key to preventing denials, winning appeals, and preventing accusations of fraudulent activity by governmental agencies (e.g., Office of Inspector General, Recovery Audit Contractors). CMS points out that clear and concise health information documentation is critical to the quality of patient care and is required for payment of services rendered. Documentation is also necessary to support the medical necessity of services and to ensure compliance with regulatory requirements. Healthcare organizations must have policies and procedures in place to maintain the integrity of the health record.

## DOCUMENTATION REQUIREMENTS WHEN ASSIGNING E/M CODES

When a physician selects the physical examination component of an evaluation and management (E/M) code, he/she must provide documentation to support that selection. To aid in this selection process, the AMA has outlined the documentation requirements for the key components of an E/M code (e.g., history, physical examination, and medical decision making). The documentation requirements for the physical examination are divided into four types of examinations. They are problem-focused exam, expanded problem-focused exam, detailed exam, and comprehensive exam.

Further explanation of each exam is as follows:

| Type of Exam | Extent of Exam | Assessment Results |
| --- | --- | --- |
| Problem-focused | Limited to an affected body part or organ | 1 to 5 structures or functions of the body part/organ |
| Expanded problem-focused | Limited to an affected body part or organ | 6 structures or functions of 1 or more body systems |
| Detailed | Extended exam of body areas | At least 2 structures or functions in 6 organ systems OR at least 12 structures or functions in 2 or more organ systems |
| Comprehensive | Multisystem exam | At least 2 structures or functions in 9 organ systems OR all structures or functions in the affected organ system AND at least 1 structure or function of the remaining organ systems |

## ROLE REGARDING CPT CODE ASSIGNMENTS

When services are provided in a physician's office or clinic, the CPT code will be selected by the physician from an encounter form or superbill. The coder or biller is responsible for transferring the selected codes from the encounter form onto the insurance claim form. However, before assigning the code onto the claim form, the coder/biller must review the medical record documentation to ensure the code is supported. Inevitably, there will be occasions where a higher or lower level E/M code should have been selected, and it is the coder's/biller's responsibility to verify the accuracy of the selected code. The process differs in the hospital outpatient setting, where it is the coder's responsibility to select the appropriate CPT code based upon the physician's documentation.

## MEDICARE'S REQUIREMENTS FOR E/M SERVICES

Medicare funds are protected under the Social Security Act. Section 1862(a)(1)(A) of the Act stipulates that Medicare will only reimburse for services that are reasonable and necessary. It is the healthcare provider's responsibility to bill the appropriate evaluation and management (E/M) code. The healthcare provider must not bill a higher level E/M code for services that were rendered at a lower level. In order to support the codes billed, it is imperative that the healthcare provider's documentation be accurate and thorough, so that there is no question of fraudulent activity. Section 1833(e) of the Social Security Act prohibits payment for any code that is not supported with acceptable documentation.

## Code Sequencing According to Healthcare Setting

### PRINCIPAL DIAGNOSIS

The principal (PDX) is one of the most important code assignments a coder can select. In many instances, the PDX will be the "driver" behind the diagnosis-related group (DRG) (also known as "disease groupings") selection. Of course, secondary diagnoses (SDX), which may be designated as a major complication or comorbidity (MCC) or a complication/comorbidity (CC), can also impact the DRG assignment. Regardless of which diagnoses (or sometimes even procedure) code is the "driver" behind the DRG assignment, the PDX is still one of upmost importance for correct selection. The PDX is defined by the UHDDS as the condition established *after study* to be responsible for causing the patient's admission to the hospital. There are many coding guidelines to consider when determining the PDX, and its assignment can be a source of disagreements between coders and auditors (internal and/or external). Therefore, it is essential a coder review the entire medical record for the complete picture of the patient's case and determine what occasioned the admission *after study*.

### PROPERLY SEQUENCING ICD-10-CM CODES FOR AN INPATIENT

The sequencing of diagnostic codes is key to accurate diagnosis-related group (DRG) assignment. Code sequencing drives the selection of the principal diagnosis, which is really the most important code assignment a coder will make. Of course, the principal diagnosis must be selected at the highest level of specificity, followed by secondary diagnoses. Some secondary diagnoses are classified as complications/comorbidities (CCs) or major complications/comorbidities (MCCs). They, too, will impact the DRG assignment. The relationship between the principal and secondary diagnoses is factored into DRG grouper logic. Coders must be vigilant in reviewing all healthcare documentation in order to select and sequence all diagnoses correctly for the most compliant and financially impactful order. Of note, it is also possible for an ICD-10-PCS procedure code to impact the DRG assignment.

### RE-SEQUENCING CODES IN ICD-10

AHIMA has an established Standards of Ethical Coding that coders are expected to follow. The standards emphasize that all healthcare data elements (e.g., diagnosis codes, procedure codes) must be reported completely and accurately and supported by healthcare documentation. One standard points out that coders are not to change codes for the purpose of inappropriately increasing payment. Therefore, it is important that coders apply official coding guidelines correctly and only re-sequence the order of codes according to ICD-10 rules. Re-sequencing codes can either have a positive or negative financial impact because the DRG selection can change to a higher or lower paying rate. If documentation does not support the DRG change, the healthcare organization could be accused of upcoding for financial gain. This can place the healthcare organization at risk of being found guilty of fraudulent claim billing.

# Determining Evaluation and Management (E/M) Level

## Contribution of History and Exam to the Level of an Outpatient E/M

Before January 1, 2021, the history and physical examination of a patient were components that contributed to the leveling of an outpatient E/M. Now, CPT guidelines only require that a "medically appropriate history and/or examination" are obtained from the patient, which is determined by the provider's clinical judgment. Collection of a patient's personal, family, and social history, along with the nature of their presenting problem(s) may be done directly by the provider and/or other healthcare staff members. This information may also be collected indirectly, either by a questionnaire or by a review of previously reported data in the patient's electronic health record.

## Differences Among History Components

There are three elements that collectively contribute to the history component of an inpatient, emergency, observation, and nursing facility care E/M:

- History of present illness (HPI)
- Review of systems (ROS)
- Past medical, family, and/or social history (PFSH)

The minimum amount of information collected from the patient would level to a problem-focused exam, only requiring a brief collection of HPI. An expanded problem-focused history requires the same, but with the addition of a pertinent ROS. A detailed history documents an extended HPI, an extended ROS, and a pertinent PFSH. Lastly, a comprehensive history represents the most amount of data collected: an extended HPI, a complete ROS, and a complete PFSH.

## Differences of the 1995 and 1997 E/M Guidelines

According to the E/M guidelines issued in 1995, a provider or other healthcare professional could choose to level their examination based on a how many body areas they evaluated on a patient or based on the number of organ systems. Body areas include, but are not limited to, the abdomen, neck, and extremities. Organ systems include skin, cardiovascular, and respiratory, among others. Because many specialty providers found the 1995 guidelines to not be specific enough, the 1997 E/M guidelines were issued. The exam portion of the 1997 E/M guidelines includes 11 specialties (genitourinary, cardiovascular, eye, respiratory, etc.) in which up to 12 elements can be selected within multiple body areas. For example, instead of just selecting respiratory in the organ system of the 1995 guidelines, a provider could now select the following elements: percussion of chest, auscultation of lungs, inspection of teeth and gums, etc. However, because the 1997 guidelines were viewed as being too cumbersome, either set of guidelines are able to be used when leveling the exam portion of a medical record.

## Types of Medical Decision Making

The four types of medical decision making are straightforward, low complexity, moderate complexity, and high complexity. In order to determine which of the four types a medical note would constitute, three elements would need to be considered:

- 1) number and complexity of problems addressed
- 2) amount and/or complexity of data reviewed
- 3) risk of complications and/or morbidity or mortality

To determine which of the four types of medical decision making is supported, take the lowest of the two highest elements.

An 18-year-old male patient arrives in the ED complaining of right lower quadrant abdominal pain and vomiting. A urinalysis reveals leukocytosis; therefore, an abdominal ultrasound is ordered to rule out appendicitis. The patient will be admitted and started on IV fluids.

| Element | Decision Level |
| --- | --- |
| Number and complexity of problems addressed | Moderate complexity |
| Amount and/or complexity of data reviewed | Limited/low complexity |
| Risk of complications and/or morbidity or mortality | Moderate complexity |

## PROBLEM(S) ADDRESSED IN THE MEDICAL DECISION-MAKING RISK TABLE

When determining the four types of medical decision making, the number and complexity of problem(s) addressed should be considered first. Simply listing a diagnosis in the assessment, stating that a different physician and/or practice is evaluating it, and/or only issuing a referral for a diagnosis does not constitute a provider addressing or managing it. On the other hand, a provider does not necessarily need to be actively treating an illness in order for it to qualify as being addressed or managed. For example, if a physician is treating a patient for pneumonia by issuing a prescription for amoxicillin, but also had to consider a potential drug interaction with the patient's long-term anticoagulant due to chronic atrial fibrillation, both illnesses should be credited to the provider.

## DATA REVIEWED IN THE MEDICAL DECISION-MAKING RISK TABLE

When determining the four types of medical decision making, the amount and/or complexity of data reviewed should be considered second. The data are divided into three subcategories:

- Each individual test, document, or independent historian(s)
- Independent interpretation of the tests
- Discussion of management or test interpretation

If the provider is separately reporting a test or its interpretation, the ordering and/or reviewing of such a test cannot be credited in the amount and/or complexity of data reviewed when leveling an E/M. The consideration of this element begins with E/M codes 99203 and 99213, in which at least one entire subcategory must be met. For E/M codes 99204 and 99214, just one entire subcategory must also be met; however, three individual tests or documents are required to fulfill one subcategory instead of just two. Lastly, for E/M codes 99205 and 99215, at least two entire subcategories must be met.

## COMPLICATIONS AND/OR MORBIDITY OR MORTALITY IN THE MEDICAL DECISION-MAKING RISK TABLE

The risk of complications and/or morbidity or mortality is the final element to be reviewed when determining the four types of medical decision making. The American Medical Association defines risk as "the probability and/or consequences of an event." Examples are provided on the E/M audit worksheets as a guide. For example, if a patient is advised to rest or gargle, the risk of complication or death resulting from such an action is considered minimal (99202 or 99212). On the other hand, if surgical intervention is recommended and risks are discussed, the likelihood of complications is considered high, driving this element alone to equate to a 99205 or 99215, depending on if the patient is new or established.

## SCENARIO

A 78-year-old man is seen in the office for a medication renewal. He has a history of type 2 diabetes and hypertension. He has been compliant with medication and has no complaints. A comprehensive exam was performed with no abnormal findings. Lab requisition will be given to assess his A1C level. Current medications will be renewed at the current dosage, and advise patient to follow up in 3 months, unless blood work comes back abnormal or the patient develops other symptoms.

The level of medical decision making for this scenario is moderate. The patient has type 2 diabetes and hypertension, which are two of the most common chronic health conditions. Other common illnesses that are considered to be chronic include asthma, heart disease, arthritis, and osteoporosis. Because the patient has been compliant with his medication and the physical exam was normal, "two or more stable chronic illnesses" can be selected from the **moderate** box within the "number and complexity of problems addressed" in the medical decision-making audit tool. Next, "review the amount and/or complexity of data to review and analyze." Because the provider ordered just one outside lab to test the patient's glucose level, this section would be considered **minimal**. Third, determine the risk of the patient's current illnesses. The physician decided to maintain the current prescription and dosage; therefore, this would be considered **moderate**. Finally, the overall medical decision-making score is obtained by taking the lowest of the two highest boxes. In this scenario, the two highest boxes are the same, so the medical decision making is considered moderate.

## DETERMINING THE LEVEL OF SERVICE OF AN OUTPATIENT E/M BASED ON TIME

CPT defines a new patient as one who has not received care from a provider or other qualified healthcare professional within the same practice in the exact same specialty and subspecialty within the past 3 years. An established patient is one who has previously received care by a provider or other qualified healthcare professional in the same practice in the exact same specialty and subspecialty within the past 3 years. To level an E/M based on time, the provider or other qualified healthcare professional must document in the medical record the total time they personally spent on the care of the patient on the date of primary service.

| Code | Description |
|---|---|
| 99202 | 15–29 minutes |
| 99203 | 30–44 minutes |
| 99204 | 45–59 minutes |
| 99205 | 60–74 minutes |
| 99211 | a short encounter that may not require the presence of a physician (i.e., a blood pressure check) |
| 99212 | 10–19 minutes |
| 99213 | 20–29 minutes |
| 99214 | 30–39 minutes |
| 99215 | 40–54 minutes |
| +99417 | each additional 15 minutes of total time, listed as an add-on code to CPT codes 99215 and 99205 |

## LEVELING AN OUTPATIENT E/M BASED ON TIME

Leveling an E/M based on time includes total face-to-face time spent on the care of the patient on the date of the primary service, such as performing a medically appropriate physical examination and history, counseling and/or educating the patient, family, and/or caregiver, and management of the presenting illness(es), including issuing referrals, prescriptions, tests, or procedures. The total time also includes non–face-to-face time spent on the care of the patient on the date of the primary service. Examples include when a provider or other qualified healthcare professional must communicate to another healthcare professional, reviewing tests or history prior to the patient's encounter, and/or documenting clinical information in the health record following the patient's encounter. Time spent traveling to the office, teaching that is not related to a specific patient, and performing procedures that are being separately reported are not allowed to be included in the total time.

## Using Appropriate Modifiers

### MODIFIERS

Modifiers are two-digit alphabetical, numerical, or alphanumerical characters that are appended to CPT and HCPCS II codes. They are used indicate anatomical locations (i.e., LT indicates the left side), the health status of a patient (i.e., P1 represents a normal, healthy patient), determine who rendered medical care (i.e., GC reports a service rendered by a resident under the oversight of a physician), the method by which a service was rendered (i.e., 95 indicates that a service was rendered via video), and report that a medical service or procedure was modified in some way, in some cases due to special circumstances (i.e., 57 indicates that an E/M resulted in a decision for surgery).

### MODIFIER 25 VS. MODIFIER 59

The main difference between modifiers 25 and 59 are the procedural codes that they are attached to. Modifier 25 is used to report a "significant, separately identifiable evaluation and management service by the same physician or other qualified healthcare professional on the same day of the procedure or other service." As an example, 99213-25, 69210 could be reported in the following scenario: during a follow-up for diabetes, the patient was found to have impacted cerumen, which was removed on the same day. Modifier 59 is used when two procedures (other than E/M services) are performed on the same day and by the same provider that are not normally reported together. As an example, two separate lesions differing in size are removed from a patient's back thorax. In this scenario, report 11402, 11401-59.

### MODIFIER 52 VS. MODIFIER 53

Modifier 52 is appended on surgical procedures for which anesthesia is not required, to indicate that a procedure was partially reduced or eliminated after the patient was prepared and/or brought into the surgical room. The provider may expect to partially reduce the procedure, or the patient may decide to cancel it prior to its completion. For example, if a 13-year-old patient is only having one tonsil removed, report 42826-52. Modifier 52 may also be used on radiology services, for which no other code exists to report what service was rendered. Modifier 53 is appended on procedures that may or may not require anesthesia, to indicate that the service has been discontinued. It may be discontinued because of a change in the patient's health status or due to extenuating circumstances, such as equipment failure. For example, if a coronary artery graft repair had to be discontinued when a patient's blood pressure suddenly dropped, report 33503-53.

### MODIFIER 58 VS. MODIFIER 78

Modifier 58 is used on a staged or related procedure performed by the same physician during the 10- or 90-day postoperative period. Keywords when reporting modifier 58 would include planned, anticipated, or staged. Modifier 78 is used on an unplanned procedure performed by the same physician following an initial procedure for a related procedure during the 10- or 90-day postoperative period. For example, if a patient develops an infection within the 90-day postoperative period following a hip replacement that requires the removal of the hip prosthesis, report 27091-78. Reporting the unplanned procedure does not extend the postoperative period of the initial procedure.

# Reimbursement Methodologies

## Code Sequencing and Payer Specific Guidelines

### RE-SEQUENCING ICD-10-CM CODES FOR OPTIMAL REIMBURSEMENT

When assigning ICD-10-CM codes for an inpatient encounter, there are occasions wherein it would be appropriate to re-sequence the codes in order to obtain optimal reimbursement. This usually occurs when the ICD-10 Official Coding Guideline for selection of the principal diagnosis is referenced (Section IIC). The Section IIC guideline is used when two or more diagnoses equally meet the definition for the principal diagnosis. Of course, the coder must ensure that both diagnoses were determined to be the cause of the admission and both were treated therapeutically or "worked up" with diagnostic procedures. If all of these factors are met, then either diagnosis may be sequenced first. An example of when this guideline could be applied follows: A patient was admitted with exacerbation of chronic obstructive pulmonary disease (COPD) and acute on chronic diastolic heart failure. Both conditions were treated with intravenous medications, oxygen therapy, and respiratory therapy. Since both diagnoses were the reason for the patient's admission and both were treated equally, either one could be selected as the principal diagnosis. Subsequently, the one associated with a higher weighted DRG should be chosen as the principal diagnosis.

### IMPACT OF DRG WEIGHTS ON REIMBURSEMENT

Diagnosis-related groups, or DRGs, as they are better known, are a group of related conditions/diseases that are a component of the inpatient prospective payment system (IPPS). The IPPS is a payment system set forth by the Social Security Act for Medicare Part A recipients that reimburses healthcare entities for their operating expenses associated with the provision of acute care inpatient stays. Each DRG has its own unique weight based on the average amount of resources used to treat patients that fall into that category. Those conditions that are most costly will be categorized in a higher weighted DRG. To calculate a DRG reimbursement rate, a standardized amount for labor and non-labor components, wage index factor, cost of living adjustment, and earnings by occupational category are all calculated into the reimbursement rate.

### POA INDICATOR

The purpose of the present on admission (POA) indicator is to indicate which conditions are present at admission and which conditions develop during an inpatient admission. One of the following five POA indicators must be reported with all codes: Y – yes, the condition/disease was present on admission; N – no, the condition/disease was not present on admission; U – unknown, documentation is insufficient to determine; W – clinically undetermined by provider whether present on admission; and, or 1 – exempt from reporting. A POA indicator of N or U may impact the reimbursement of codes because this designation would indicate a "hospital-acquired conditions" (HAC). POA indicator data can be used for multiple purposes: financial, research, and quality of care.

### IDENTIFYING HACS

A hospital-acquired condition (HAC) is an unfavorable condition (e.g., an infection, development of a decubitus ulcer) that occurs during the hospitalization and adversely affects the patient's health and course of treatment. Another way to understand HACs is to think of them as complications or nosocomial infections/conditions. The Deficit Reduction Act of 2005 requires the reporting of conditions that are of a high cost or high volume and that could have been potentially prevented by following guidance from evidence-based outcomes. A current list of HACs is maintained by the

Centers for Medicare and Medicaid Services (CMS) and can be accessed through CMS.gov. The ultimate goal in identifying HACs is to provide an incentive to hospitals to reduce HACs. CMS has instituted a HAC Reduction Program (HACRP). HACRP adjusts payments to healthcare entities that rank in the worst-performing quartile of all hospitals. Nationwide, hospitals can be compared online through the Medicare.gov Hospital Compare site.

## EFFECT OF COMBINATION CODING ON SEQUENCING OF CODES

Combination codes are required for some disease processes in ICD-10-CM coding. Combination codes are recognized as a single code that represents two disease processes. They can also represent one diagnosis with an associated symptom, or one diagnosis with an associated complication. The purpose behind having combination codes is to reduce the overall number of codes assigned for a case as well as reduce any sequencing problems. In an improvement from ICD-9-CM, combination codes in ICD-10-CM have simplified sequencing dilemmas. Some examples of combination codes are:

| Disease Process | Disease Process | Symptom | Complication | ICD-10 Combination Code |
|---|---|---|---|---|
| Cholelithiasis with... | Cholecystitis | N/A | N/A | K80.10 |
| Diabetes with... | N/A | N/A | Gastroparesis | E10.43 |
| Acute cystitis with... | N/A | Hematuria | N/A | N30.01 |

## LINKING DIAGNOSES AND CPT CODES

It is important to remember that CPT procedural codes must be linked to a corresponding ICD-10-CM diagnosis code. Failure to link the two codes will most likely result in a medical necessity denial of the claim by the payer. The ICD-10-CM code links the diagnosis to the treatment represented by the CPT code. The outpatient claim form allows for more than one ICD-10-CM code to be included; however, many payers will only notice the first-listed ICD-10-CM code. Therefore, it is critical that the coder ensure the diagnosis code has a matching procedural code. In doing so, denials management is an easier task for the revenue cycle team.

## NUMBER OF CPT CODES THAT MAY BE LINKED TO ONE DIAGNOSIS CODE

Every CPT procedural code must be linked to a corresponding diagnosis code. The selected diagnosis code should support the medical necessity of the procedure. To know if the diagnosis code is supportive, one would need to reference CMS's national coverage determination (NCD) or the local coverage determination (LCD) to see if the diagnosis code is listed there as a covered diagnosis. There will be occasions when one diagnosis code will support multiple CPT procedural codes. This is an acceptable coding practice. For example, an ankle fracture may require multiple procedures to stabilize the joint. The diagnosis code for ankle fracture would support all procedures performed for the joint stabilization, and thus all procedures would be reimbursed.

# DRG and APC Methodologies

## DRG

### STRUCTURE OF DRGS

Diagnosis-related groups (DRGs) represent categories of patients who are medically related based upon their diagnoses/conditions and treatment of the diagnoses/conditions. Another factor of similarity between the categories is the lengths of inpatient stays. The patients categorized in the various DRGs require similar amounts of resources related to costs. DRGs are hierarchical, meaning that they belong to major diagnostic categories (MDCs) that represent body systems. In 2007, DRGs were replaced with Medicare Severity DRGs (MS-DRGs); therefore, replacing the 538 DRGs with 745 new MS-DRGs. (This number varies internationally.) The MS-DRG system is a 3-tiered system that offers choices pertaining to major complications/comorbidities (MCC), complications/comorbidities (CC), and no complication/comorbidity (non-CC).

## STRUCTURE OF MDCS

Major diagnostic categories (MDCs) were established for the purpose of categorizing patients according to diseases and disorders by body system. MDCs are either medically or surgically structured. Medical MDCs are further divided into diagnosis-related groups (DRGs) that are structured based upon principal diagnoses. Surgical MDCs are further divided into DRGs based upon surgical procedure(s) performed. In 2016, there are 25 MDCs. An MDC decision tree or algorithm will consider various elements to determine the correct DRG as noted in the following example:

- Was an operative procedure performed?
    - Yes – What type of surgery?
        - Major surgery?
            - DRG __
        - Minor surgery?
            - DRG __
    - No – What is the principal diagnosis?
        - Neoplasm?
            - MCC/CC?
            - DRG __
        - Specific conditions related to body system?
            - MCC/CC?
            - DRG __

## IPPS

The inpatient prospective payment system (IPPS) is Medicare's payment system for acute care inpatient hospital stays, specifically Medicare Severity Diagnosis Related Groups (MS-DRGs). MS-DRGs have been around since 2007, and provide higher reimbursement for acute care hospitals treating more severely ill patients than those that treat less severely ill patients. If an acute care hospital serves a disproportionate number of low-income patients, that hospital will receive an add-on payment, known as the Disproportionate Share Hospital (DHS) payment. If the hospital is an approved teaching hospital, an add-on payment will be provided also. There are other factors under IPPS wherein hospitals may receive additional payments (e.g., new technologies, sole community hospitals). IPPS is regulated by CMS and is updated annually in order to stay compliant with the Affordable Care Act. The changes are published annually in the Federal Register.

## APC

### STRUCTURE OF APCS

Ambulatory Payment Classifications, or APCs, is Medicare's payment methodology for outpatient services. One could describe it as the "DRG" system for outpatient services. APCs are an outpatient prospective payment system (OPPS) for hospitals only. They have no impact upon physician's services as those services are reimbursed under the Medicare Physician Fee Schedule. Medicare will only issue an APC payment when the patient is discharged from an outpatient service, such as the emergency department or a provider-based clinic. If the patient is admitted, no APC payment is rendered because at that point, the patient's payment is made from the inpatient prospective payment system (IPPS). APCs are similar to DRGs in that services are grouped together according to resource utilization and cost.

## APC PAYMENTS
### HOSPITAL SERVICES THAT ARE COVERED UNDER APC PAYMENT

Ambulatory Payment Classification (APC) payments apply to services rendered in an outpatient setting. These outpatient services may be rendered in an outpatient surgery setting, outpatient clinic setting, emergency departments, and/or observation services. APC payments are not only applicable to therapeutic services, but they also are applicable for diagnostic services, such as radiology, or for drug infusion services, such as chemotherapy infusions. It is important to know that APC payments do not apply to physician services because those services are reimbursed under the Medicare Physician Fee Schedule. APC payment amounts are calculated by multiplying a service's relative weight against the "conversion factor." The APC conversion factor for 2016 is $73.728. The APC payment amount is adjusted according to each hospital's geographical location.

### EFFECT OF ICD-10-CM CODES ON APC PAYMENTS

ICD-10-CM codes do not affect APC payments in a *direct* manner. The diagnostic codes are not used to determine facility reimbursement. They are, however, important from a medical necessity standpoint, and in that way, they *indirectly* affect APC payments. In other words, without an appropriate and/or approved ICD-10-CM diagnosis code to establish the medical necessity of the outpatient services, APC reimbursement will not occur. Local coverage determinations (LCDs) and/or national coverage determinations (NCDs) provide the necessary guidance for coders to know whether or not an ICD-10-CM diagnosis code is considered a medically necessary diagnosis for each procedure.

### EFFECT OF PACKAGING OF ITEMS AND SERVICES ON APC PAYMENTS

Packaging of items and services in the Outpatient Prospective Payment System (OPPS) is commonly noted in Ambulatory Payment Classifications (APCs). Within each APC, at a minimum, the following services are packaged or included:

- Supplies
- Ancillary services
- Anesthesia
- Operating room and recovery room use
- Lab tests
- Implants/Devices
- Drugs (e.g., radiological drugs, contrasts)
- Imaging services and their interpretation

These services are not separately payable because they are considered to be integral to the service/procedure. Coders must follow appropriate coding guidelines when deciding if a service is packaged or if it can be unbundled and billed separately.

## LOCATING APC PAYMENT TABLES ON CMS.GOV

Ambulatory Payment Classifications (APCs) are updated annually. The updated payment rates are posted for general public knowledge on the CMS.gov site. To locate the table, there are several steps to follow. They are:

- Navigate to CMS.gov
- Select the Medicare tab
- Under the "Medicare Fee-for-Service Payment" section, select Hospital Outpatient PPS
- In the toolbar on the left side, select "Addendum A and Addendum B"
- Select the most current "Release Date"
- Select the related link for Addendum A or B
- Accept the license for use of CPT
- Open the zip file
- Open the corresponding Excel spreadsheet

The Excel spreadsheet will contain the most current APC payment rates per CPT code.

# NCCI Edits

## NATIONAL CORRECT CODING INITIATIVE

The National Correct Coding Initiative (NNCCI) was developed by CMS for the purpose of encouraging correct coding methodologies nationwide. NCCI is applicable to Part B claims only. Healthcare entities can assess their coding accuracy prior to submitting a Part B claim and thus potentially prevent an inappropriate payment and/or a denial. NCCI edits (also known as Procedure-to-Procedure [PTP] code pair edits) can provide the guidance needed to assess coding accuracy. Additionally, there are Medically Unlikely Edits (MUEs) that identify the maximum number of units that can be billed for a single code. All of these measures aid the coder/biller in preventing inappropriate code combinations.

## MEDICARE CODE EDITS FOR ICD-10-PCS CODES

For ICD-10-CM/PCS codes, Medicare has code edits in place to assist with coding accuracy. Some of the Medicare Code Edits (MCE) are as follows:

- Invalid diagnosis or procedure code – Each code is compared against a table of valid codes, and if a submitted code does not match a code in the table, it is considered invalid.
- Age conflict – If a diagnosis or procedure code is clinically impossible, an edit identifies the conflict. There are four recognized age groups in ICD-10 – newborn, pediatric, adult, and maternity.
- Gender/Sex conflict with the code.
- Non-covered procedure – Medicare does not provide coverage for all procedures.
- Procedure with limited coverage - Medicare limits reimbursement for some procedures that have associated extraordinary costs.

## RESOLVING NCCI EDITS

Certified coders, who are knowledgeable in proper coding methodologies, should be involved in the workflow process of reconciling any National Correct Coding Initiative (NCCI) edits. An NCCI edit is an indication that at least one code in the code pair is incorrect. Therefore, in such a scenario, the coder can reference the medical record documentation and determine what coding corrections are needed. Coders may also be able to identify any inaccurate charges assigned by the various hospital departments, or they may be able to make recommendations for chargemaster changes in order to remain in compliance with coding regulations.

## MODIFIERS THAT ARE ALLOWED WITH THE NCCI EDITS

Modifiers may be appended to a CPT code so that a CCI edit can be bypassed. Bypassing an edit, however, should only be done if the clinical documentation supports the addition of the modifier. The NCCI edit table will indicate whether the application of a modifier is allowed or not (0 = no modifiers allowed, 1 = modifiers allowed). Anatomical modifiers (e.g., F1, F2, etc.), surgical modifiers (e.g., 25, 58, etc.), and other modifiers (e.g., XE, XP, etc.) are allowed, again depending upon guidance per code in the edit table.

# Coverage Determinations

## NCD AND LCD

National coverage determinations (NCDs) are published by Medicare for the purpose of noting what services or procedures will be covered by Medicare. An NCD is mandated at the national level for all fiscal intermediaries and Medicare Administrative Contractors (MACs) to follow. Local coverage determinations (LCD) are established by each MAC for the purpose of establishing further guidance beyond the NCD or by providing guidance in the absence of an NCD. LCDs are applicable to the corresponding MAC's jurisdiction. Both NCDs and LCDs are primarily intended to provide medical necessity guidance. CMS.gov maintains a Medicare Coverage Database wherein one can locate NCDs and LCDs, whether they are current, retired, or proposed.

## CMS CREATING AN NCD

The Centers for Medicare and Medicaid Services (CMS) develops national coverage determinations (NCDs) when there is a need to provide coverage for new healthcare technologies or procedures or when there is a need to consider an existing procedure as being beneficial for national Medicare coverage. The process of developing a new NCD usually takes between 6 and 9 months and involves assessment of the national coverage request, advisory committee reviews, staff reviews, draft decisions, public comments, and final decision implementation. Of interest, a local coverage determination (LCD) can become an NCD if approved to be adopted nationally.

## LOCATING AN NCD/LCD ONLINE

CMS.gov/Medicare-coverage-database is one of the quickest ways to locate a national coverage determination (NCD) or a local coverage determination (LCD). All NCDs and LCDs, regardless of status (e.g., active, retired, future, or proposed) are maintained in this database. Searches can be done by reviewing the alphabetic index, conducting a search for the NCD/LCD title (if known), or by searching according to geographic region. Once the desired NCD/LCD is located, either the content will be available for review immediately or one will need to select the link to the pdf file.

## MEDICAL NECESSITY

The basic concept of medical necessity is that invasive procedures and diagnostic studies should only be performed when they are medically necessary. Medical necessity is the deciding factor as to whether or not a payer will reimburse the healthcare entity for the expenditures associated with the procedure or testing. There must be a clear medical reason for a procedure to be performed. A diagnosis must support the procedure as well as provide further evidence of the medical necessity. NCDs and LCDs will outline medical necessity criteria. If Medicare has determined that a procedure is not medically necessary, the patient must be notified of the decision through an advance beneficiary notice (ABN), which alerts the patient to their associated costs.

## ABN

Advance beneficiary notice (ABN) (of Noncoverage) is a tool used to notify traditional Medicare beneficiaries that Medicare will most likely deny payment of certain services. This notice allows the beneficiary the opportunity to make an informed decision about whether or not to proceed with the service. If they choose to proceed with the service, it could be an out-of-pocket expense for the beneficiary. There are three occurrences when an ABN is required:

- When the service does not meet medical necessity guidelines
- When the service may only be paid a limited number of times within a specific time frame
- When the service is for research purposes

It is important to understand that the ABN *must* be provided before the service is undertaken. It is never appropriate to issue an ABN when the Medicare patient is in an emergency situation because this would conflict with the Emergency Medical Treatment & Labor Act (EMTALA) regulations. Once the emergency situation is stabilized, issuance of an ABN may be appropriate.

# Claim Forms

### LIFE CYCLE OF A CLAIM

The life cycle of a claim begins with the creation of a patient encounter, whether through the emergency department, outpatient services, or an inpatient admission. Services are then rendered for the patient, and charges associated with the services are entered into the patient accounting system. After discharge of the patient from inpatient or outpatient status and upon review of documentation, appropriate ICD-10 codes are assigned. Editing and correction of the charges and codes on the claim are performed prior to billing the claim. The claim will be processed through a clearinghouse. Following this step, either payment will be made by the payer(s), or if denials are rendered, appeals may be necessary. A remittance advice (RA) or an explanation of benefits (EOB) will be provided by the payer to the healthcare entity. Collections of funds may also be necessary as a last step in the claim's life cycle process.

### PAYER MATCHING

When a claim is submitted to an insurance carrier by the healthcare entity, the claim will be scrubbed, which means it will be checked for errors. Once any identified errors are corrected, the claim will be forwarded onto the payer for review. In order to ensure the claim goes to the correct payer, it must go through a process known as payer matching. Payer matching begins when a healthcare provider enrolls with a clearinghouse, and at that time, the payer is matched to the provider through the assignment of a payer identification (ID) number. This payer ID number instructs the clearinghouse as to which payer should receive the claim.

### COORDINATION OF BENEFITS

When an individual is covered by more than one insurance plan, guidelines pertaining to coordination of benefits (COB) will instruct healthcare providers as to which insurance carrier to bill as the primary payer and which insurance carrier(s) to bill as the secondary or tertiary payer. The COB process ensures that claims are paid correctly through the coordination of the payment process. The COB process also transmits claims paid by the primary payer onto the secondary payer for payment of the balance. The COB process also ensures that between all payers only up to 100% of the claim is reimbursed, which eliminates any possibility of duplicate payments.

## Forms Used for Submitting Claims

In healthcare, there are two forms used for claims submission. They are the UB-04 and the CMS-1500. The UB-04 is a universal claim form that is used by hospitals, critical access hospitals, hospices, home health agencies, outpatient rehab facilities, end-stage renal disease facilities, skilled nursing facilities, etc. The UB-04 is widely accepted by nearly all insurance companies. It is maintained by the National Uniform Billing Committee (NUBC). There are general guidelines for correct completion of its 81 fields, also known as form locators (FL). The CMS-1500 form is maintained by the Centers for Medicare and Medicaid Services (CMS). Its use is required for reporting provider/physician services. It, too, has general guidelines for correct completion of its 33 fields.

## Consequences of Filing a Claim with Falsified Information

The most obvious consequence of filing a claim with incorrect or falsified information would be rejection of the claim and/or denial of the payment by the insurance payer. On a more serious note, individuals and entities can be penalized for filing false claims. It is illegal to submit claims for payment to Medicare or Medicaid that are knowingly false or fraudulent. The penalties can start with fines ranging between $5,000 and $11,000 per claim, and penalties can even lead to imprisonment for felony convictions under federal and/or state laws.

## Submitting a Claim Form for Non-Covered Charges

The CMS has specific instructions on how to file claims for non-covered charges. The Medicare beneficiary must have been notified that the services would not be paid by Medicare through the process of issuing an advance beneficiary notice (ABN). The ABN allows the beneficiary the opportunity to make an informed decision about whether or not to proceed with the service. If the choice is to proceed, the services are considered to be non-covered, and completion of the claim must be completed as follows. For inpatient (IP) claims, the non-covered services may be reported on a no-pay claim, Type of Bill 110. For outpatient claims, the non-covered services must be appended with a modifier GA or GX. Modifier GA indicates a mandatory ABN was issued, and modifier GX indicates a voluntary ABN was issued. When CMS receives claims containing these indicators, that line item on the claim representing the non-covered charge is automatically denied. The financial liability shifts to the beneficiary.

# Communicating with Financial Departments

## Relevant Financial Reports That Are Relevant to Both Coding and Patient Financial Services

Effective communication between the coding department and patient financial services (PFS) is essential to revenue cycle operations in a healthcare institution. There are primarily three areas wherein the two departments must collaborate. One of the primary tools used by the coding or health information management (HIM) department is the DNFB monitoring report. DNFB is the acronym for "discharged not final billed." By monitoring this report, old accounts and/or high dollar accounts can be addressed quickly. Another area of collaboration between the two departments would be in dealing with medical necessity. Patient financial employees check a claim for medical necessity prior to submission of the bill, and coders are key to obtaining additional information from physicians to support medical necessity. NCCI edits are a third area that requires collaboration in order to resolve edit conflicts. Coders can resolve edits by removing charges and/or correcting codes.

## REVENUE CYCLE MANAGEMENT

Revenue cycle management in healthcare is a three-part process. It involves management of the healthcare institution's claims processing, payment processing, and revenue generation. The revenue cycle begins at the point of determining patient eligibility, collecting the patient's copay and/or deductible, correct coding of claims, correct charging of services, tracking claims between the provider and the payer, collecting payments, and claims denial management. Two other factors impact revenue for a healthcare entity: provider/physician productivity and patient volume (admissions/ discharges/ transfers).

## PAYMENT MODELS FOR WHICH THE CODING AND FINANCIAL SERVICES' DEPARTMENTS MUST BE FAMILIAR

Obtaining reimbursement for healthcare services is a complex process. Therefore, it is imperative that the coding department and the financial services' (or revenue cycle) department communicate efficiently and effectively in order to obtain maximum reimbursement. There are several different payment models in the healthcare arena currently. The most well-known payment model is the traditional fee-for-service model. This model requires payers to reimburse each service performed. Value-based delivery care is making changes in reimbursement methodologies. This model will move away from the traditional fee-for-service model. Accountable care organizations (ACOs) are a type of value-based delivery care, wherein a large health system shares its savings by managing patients' health for less money. Incentivized payment models reward physicians for meeting certain quality and efficiency goals. Payment bundling and payment per case (e.g., DRG) continue to be popular methods of reimbursement.

# Claim Denials

## COMMON TYPES OF CLAIM DENIALS

Insurance claim denials are an expected occurrence in healthcare revenue cycle management. Some of the most common claim denials and an explanation are as follows:

| Type of Denial | Explanation |
| --- | --- |
| Technical | Denials may occur because of a problem with claims processing |
| Logic-based | Denials may occur when an ICD-10-CM or CPT code does not match a PCS Code. |
| Unspecified codes | ICD-10 coding allows for more code specificity, and unspecified codes raise red flags with payers. |
| Medical necessity | Denials may occur if medical necessity conditions are not met according to NCDs and LCDs. |
| Insurance eligibility | Denials may occur when the provider bills the wrong insurance payer. |
| Modifiers | Denials are likely to occur with modifier -25 or -59 as these two modifiers are commonly misused. |

## TRACKING DENIALS

Part of the revenue cycle management process is to track insurance payer denials and trend the reasons for the denials so that future denials can be prevented. Healthcare entities should use certain tools for the purpose of tracking denials. A claim denial spreadsheet can be used to track the reasons for denials, follow-up status, identify areas responsible for denials, and show impact on income. Dashboards are useful to display department-specific data compared against benchmarks.

Trending of data can be incorporated into the dashboards as well. Denial tracking by payer is another useful tool. One can identify and quantify such data for trending purposes.

## ADJUDICATION

Adjudication in the revenue cycle management world is a process in which submitted claims are evaluated by the payer for validity and determination of whether payment will be rendered or not. It is during the adjudication process that a claim will either be accepted, denied, or rejected. Accepted means that the payer has decided the claim is valid, but the payer may not reimburse the claim in full. They are required to process the claim according to the subscriber's plan (e.g., an 80/20 plan). A denied claim, of course, means the payer has found reason to refuse payment for the services rendered (e.g., failure to meet medical necessity). A rejected claim identified during the adjudication process means that the payer has found some type of claim error. A rejected claim may be resubmitted by the provider for reconsideration.

## MEDICARE APPEALS PROCESS FOR CLAIM DENIALS

When a healthcare provider disagrees with Medicare's payment decision, an appeal may be pursued. The appeal process can be lengthy as there are five levels of appeal. Level 1 involves a redetermination process by the company who processes claims for Medicare. Level 2 involves reconsideration by a qualified independent contractor (QIC). Level 3 would be pursued if the claim needs to be presented to an administrative law judge (ALJ). If not successful at that level, the claim can be reviewed by the Medicare Appeals Council (Level 4). A final attempt for appeal can be a judicial review in a federal district court. Each level has certain requirements to follow, and time frames can be rather long (e.g., 180 days).

## CLEAN CLAIMS

For a healthcare entity to have a 100% clean claim rate would be nothing short of a miracle. The reality is there are many challenges with submitting clean claims; however, there are strategies to follow that can reduce the number of "dirty" claims and thus reduce the number of denials. One key strategy would be for a healthcare provider to scrub claims before submitting them to the clearinghouse and/or the insurance payer. Through the process of scrubbing claims, errors are identified and routed to the appropriate personnel within the healthcare entity, who can correct the errors before dropping the claim. In order for this process to be effective, it is beneficial for the healthcare provider to be familiar with all payer edits. Careful analysis of the reasons why claims are rejected by edits is beneficial to understand as well. This ties into another strategy of staying abreast of healthcare revenue trends as well as being vigilant with the ever-changing world of governmental regulations.

## APPEALING A MEDICAL CLAIM

When a medical practice or physician's office decides to appeal medical claim(s), it is always beneficial to consider the costs involved. Of course, the best way to manage costs is to ensure that a claim is clean or valid before it is billed to the payer, thus eliminating the appeal option altogether. However, denials are an inevitable reality, and thus appeals are necessary. It is estimated that the average cost of an appeal is $20 to $25 per claim. Of course, the costs rise with each appeal. There are times an appeal might not be cost effective. For example, if the appeal is $25 and the cost of the service was only $15, the practice will lose $10 by pursuing an appeal. Therefore, management should develop policies and procedures pertaining to appropriate appeal processes.

## PROPER TRAINING AND UP-TO-DATE RESOURCES

One of the most critical steps a healthcare provider can conduct is to ensure that all revenue cycle resources are current. This requires updating of resources at least annually, and for some resources (e.g., chargemaster), updating may be more frequent. Obviously, the most current version of ICD-10 and CPT codes must be current. With the transition to ICD-10 from ICD-9 on October 1, 2015, all healthcare providers should be up-to-date with coding changes. However, it is important to note that beginning October 1, 2016, even more ICD-10 code changes are forthcoming for the fiscal year 2017. Encounter forms or charge slips should be updated when services change or charging errors are identified. The most current versions of NCDs and LCDs should be referenced, as well as the most current NCCI edits. Utilization of the most current versions of any revenue-based resource will help to reduce denials.

## Resubmitting Claims to the Payer

When a claim is rejected by Medicare, the healthcare provider may decide to resubmit the claim for reconsideration. The claim, of course, must be revised to exclude any identified errors before resubmission. The provider must also check Medicare's Common Working File (CWF) to ensure that the claim has not already been posted to a "history" status. To determine whether a historical status exists or not, the provider should access the Fiscal Intermediary Shared System (FISS) in order to generate a claims inquiry. If the claims inquiry reveals the claim has not been moved to a historical status, the provider is eligible to resubmit the corrected claim.

## Adjustments and Redeterminations

A claim adjustment means a healthcare provider has made the necessary corrections to a denied original claim, and with resubmission of the claim to the insurance carrier, the provider is canceling the original claim and replacing it with the corrected claim. The payer is able to determine if the claim is not the original by noting the "Type of Bill" (TOB) field on the claim. For example, an original inpatient claim will be referenced as a TOB 131, and a resubmitted claim will be referenced as TOB 137. The redetermination is a decision made by the payer upon receipt of the adjusted claim. The payer will review each charge on the claim, and if all is correct, the payer will issue a favorable decision to reimburse the provider for services rendered.

# Communicating Physicians to Clarify Documentation

## Physician Query Policies

Physician queries are an integral part of clinical documentation improvement (CDI) programs in healthcare institutions today. In order to standardize methods for physician query processes, query policies are recommended. Effective policies should establish query guidelines pertaining to the 4 "Ws" – who (e.g., which physician is responsible for providing clarity), what (e.g., which diagnosis or procedure is unclear), when (e.g., when is a query needed), and why (e.g., is documentation unclear or conflicting?). Policies should also address any compliance-related issues (e.g., avoidance of leading a physician to the selection of a desired diagnosis). Query policies should also explain appropriate means of following up on unanswered queries.

## Promoting Clinical Documentation Improvement Opportunities

Physicians are sometimes resistant when it comes to improving their documentation, primarily because of the belief that it entails more work for them to complete. However, there are effective ways to promote clinical documentation improvement among physicians. Some examples are:

- Communicate that good clinical documentation is instrumental in supporting quality initiatives and improved patient outcomes.
- Communicate that good clinical documentation affects quality scores related to physician contracts and reimbursement.

- Provide education that explains reimbursement concepts and how clinical documentation impacts the reimbursement methodology.
- Provide meaningful feedback and/or data to all physicians, such as most common DRGs, most common complications/comorbidities, risk of mortality scores, etc.
- Provide education pertaining to the effect of documentation problems on medical necessity.

Show examples of claim denials based on poor documentation and how better documentation would have prevented the denial.

## Hierarchical Condition Categories (HCCs) and Risk Adjustment

### HCC

HCC (Hierarchical Condition Category) is a payment model used by Medicare Advantage Plans (also known as Medicare Part C) and some other commercial managed care plans to predict the future costs of a patient over time. Estimated health costs are based on a patient's demographical location, their type of illness(es), and number of illnesses they have. The purpose of HCC is to dispense higher reimbursement rates for treating patients with chronic health conditions, with the goal of encouraging them to seek treatment and maintain their health, prior to an exacerbation or manifestation of a more serious illness. Within the HCC model, there are 19 coding categories (e.g., asthma, type 1 diabetes, substance use disorders) and 86 HCC codes (e.g., diabetes with acute complications, diabetes with chronic complications, diabetes without complications), which are comprised of more than 9,700 ICD-10-CM codes. A complete list of ICD-10-CM codes associated with current HCCs can be found on the Medicare website.

### EFFECT OF RISK ADJUSTMENT CODING ON REVENUE CYCLE

Risk adjustment coding has a direct impact on the revenue cycle for multiple reasons. The first reason has to do with a physician's documentation. If a physician thoroughly documents a patient's chronic health condition(s) and the impact it has on their health status, they are more likely to ensure quality of care and report higher levels of evaluation and management services. Additionally, specificity matters when assigning diagnosis codes. Conditions within the HCC model are assigned a risk adjustment factor (RAF). The RAF is used to determine how much a physician should be reimbursed based on how ill the patient is. For example, the RAF for a patient who suffers from diabetes is 0.118. However, if the physician documents that the patient also has chronic kidney disease, an infection, or another complication, the RAF increases to 0.368. When the RAF increases, so does reimbursement.

## Bundling and Unbundling

### UNBUNDLING CPT CODES

Unbundling occurs when certain procedures that should be reported together under one code are reported separately. Although this can increase the provider's revenue, it is illegal. For example, a lipid blood panel (CPT code 80061) consists of the following: cholesterol, serum, total (CPT code 82465); lipoprotein, direct measure, high-density cholesterol (CPT code 83718); and triglycerides (CPT code 84478). If a physician were to report the last three codes individually rather than the one CPT code for a lipid blood panel, this would be considered unbundling. The penalties of unbundling are determined by the Office of Inspector General, which range from audits, fines, imprisonment, and exclusion from Medicare and Medicaid programs.

## DETERMINING IF TWO OR MORE CPT CODES SHOULD BE BUNDLED

The National Correct Coding Initiative (NCCI) edits were created by CMS as an aid to physicians, suppliers, and hospitals to reduce incorrect payments that result from improper coding, such as unbundled procedures. Each CPT code in the NCCI edits is located next to two columns—the first column contains a different CPT code that is likely to be performed with the first, and the second column contains numbers 0, 1, or 9, called edits. Edit 0 means that the two listed procedures should never be reported together. Edit 1 means that the procedures can be reported together, but with an appropriate modifier. Lastly, edit 9 means that the edit does not apply. Referring to this list prior to billing multiple procedures can assist healthcare staff to understand when two or more CPT codes should be bundled. The complete NCCI edits can be located on the Medicare website, updated quarterly.

# Health Records and Data Content

## Retrieving Medical Records

### MEDICAL RECORD REQUEST PROCESS

Health information must be kept confidential, and the healthcare world is regulated by laws and policies that require confidentiality. In order to access patient information, release of information processes must be followed by healthcare institutions to ensure privacy is protected. An authorization to disclose personal health information (PHI) form must be submitted to the health information management (HIM) department. The form must be completed in its entirety and must designate specifically which records to release. Requestors must present government-issued photo IDs in order to validate the release. In addition to this process, healthcare institutions are providing to patients the option of accessing their PHI through web-based portals. This can provide faster access to PHI instead of waiting up to 30 days for a release through other mediums (CDs, DVDs, paper).

### RETRIEVING MEDICAL INFORMATION FROM AN ARCHIVED STATE

As patient health information ages and electronic storage space becomes limited, it is necessary for healthcare institutions to archive the information in accordance with federal and state regulatory retention guidance. Once the data are archived, they cannot be changed or deleted prior to their retention guidance, and this principle is known as immutability. The immutability of data ensures the authenticity of the data from a legal perspective. Since large amounts of archived data will need to be maintained for potentially a long period of time, storage space can be of concern; however, technology allows for intelligent compression of the data and this process reduces the amount of storage space. In order to locate archived medical information, effective indexing and searching techniques must be employed. Security of medical information data must also be incorporated into the archival process.

### CONDUCTING DATA MINING

In order to retrieve medical record or health information data, it is beneficial for a healthcare provider to implement a robust data mining program. For data mining to yield reliable results, the best practice would be for a healthcare entity to have all electronic systems and/or applications (with data collection) interfaced. Unfortunately, this concept is not a reality for most healthcare providers, but progress toward that end is being achieved. In the interim, healthcare providers should be knowledgeable of all their electronic systems, the data housed therein, and the means of gathering and reporting from all the systems. Revenue integrity data mining systems can be purchased or even built internally to maintain/manage data. Effective filtering processes can be highly effective in yielding meaningful results.

### IGPHC

Information Governance Principles of Healthcare (IGPHC) are adopted by healthcare entities to emphasize their commitment to managing complete and accurate information, which improves the quality of patient care, promotes operational efficiency, reduces risks as well as costs, and promotes compliance with regulatory agencies. Healthcare entities with effective IGPHC platforms will have implemented policies that protect/secure health information, address data aggregation for reporting purposes, and manage expanding numbers of electronic applications used in healthcare today. In addition to data security, compliance, and disposition, the information should also be "governed" to ensure data integrity, transparency, and retention. These governance principles are further explained through materials provided by the American Health Information Management Association (AHIMA).

## Analyzing Medical Records

### QUANTITATIVE ANALYSIS OF MEDICAL RECORDS

Quantitative analysis of medical records or EHR information is the process of identifying documentation deficiencies. The identified deficiencies must be resolved by the healthcare provider within a time frame of up to 30 days depending upon the type of deficiency. When analyzing for deficiencies, certain basic components must be addressed. The components are: correct patient identification on each form, presence of all required reports (as mandated by The Joint Commission, hospital bylaws, medical staff rules and regulations, CMS regulations, etc.), and authentication on all entries.

Quantitative analysis of medical records or EHR information is performed by health information personnel. The purpose of quantitative analysis is to identify documentation areas that are incomplete or inaccurate. Examples of documentation deficiencies may be a missing signature on a dictated history and physical report or a progress note, or a missing report entirely, such as a discharge summary. Regulatory guidance regarding documentation requirements provide the basis for identifying deficiencies, and health information management departments should always compose a deficiency list based on external regulations as well as bylaws and medical staff rules and regulations.

### DATA VALIDATION

Data in raw form are not as meaningful as data that have been analyzed and processed to create pertinent information for a healthcare organization. However, before data analysis can occur, there are best practices to implement. Some examples include:

- Determine the sources and types of data to capture.
- Establish and maintain a data dictionary that explains the data attributes.
- Purchase or customize tools for data collection.
- Implement data standardization formatting of templates and data fields.

Conduct routine audits of collected data to validate its integrity.

### QUALITATIVE ANALYSIS OF MEDICAL RECORDS

Qualitative analysis of medical records or health information is the process of identifying deficiencies pertaining to incomplete or inaccurate documentation. The HIM professional analyzing the documentation must understand disease processes in order to identify the deficiencies. For example, a provider may have failed to include the type of congestive heart failure (diastolic versus systolic), which is relevant information when assigning diagnostic codes. The healthcare provider can be queried to obtain clarification or further information, and it is the healthcare provider who makes the final decision that documentation is incomplete or inaccurate. Effective qualitative analysis will, in some cases, impact reimbursement as well as the quality of patient care.

## Components of a Qualitative Analysis

Qualitative analysis of medical records or health information is the process of identifying deficiencies pertaining to incomplete or inaccurate documentation. The components of qualitative analysis should include review of the following:

- Diagnostic statements for completeness (e.g., the final diagnoses in the discharge summary should include the principal diagnosis, complications, and any comorbidities that affect the hospitalization).
- Consistency in documentation by all providers so that conflicting information is avoided (e.g., physician orders for drugs should match the medication administration record).
- Justification for medical necessity throughout the patient's hospitalization (e.g., documentation must justify the course of the patient's entire stay).
- Presence of informed consent and/or consent to treatment (e.g., description of planned operation or description of potential medication side effects).

## Meaningful Use

Pursuant to passage of the American Recovery and Reinvestment Act (ARRA) of 2009, an incentive program of monetary rewards for the adoption of Health Information Technology (HIT) and Electronic Health Record (EHR) systems was initiated. In addition to adoption of HIT/EHR platforms, healthcare entities are expected to demonstrate meaningful use of the technology. Healthcare entities move through phases of implementation to ensure they are compliant with the established requirements for the electronic capture of clinical data and the exchange of information through structured formats. The overall purpose behind this incentive program is to improve the quality of patient care, improve the coordination of care, promote privacy of health information, and engage patients in their health care.

# Data Abstraction

## Data Abstraction

The purpose of data abstraction is to extract pertinent information from the medical record for multiple reasons. Standard data that should always be abstracted for statistical reasons (e.g., case mix index), reporting reasons, and compliance reasons are as follows: admit type (e.g., inpatient, outpatient, observation), admission source (e.g., transfer from another healthcare facility, emergency, scheduled), referring institution (e.g., skilled nursing facility, physician's office), discharge status (e.g., expired, alive), discharge destination (e.g., home, skilled nursing facility, hospice), cause of death (e.g., stroke, cancer, myocardial infarction), gestational age (e.g., 39 weeks), birth weight (e.g., 3,500 g), deceased date/time, admitting physician, attending physician, and consulting physicians. Data abstraction can be accomplished manually (even though this is pretty much a "thing of the past") or through the use of an HIM computer-assisted coding (CAC) system.

## HIM's Role in Information Governance

Information governance (IG) for electronic health records (EHRs) cannot be ignored despite the challenges facing healthcare organizations of large volumes of data, duplicate data, and inaccurate data. Healthcare organizations must identify key stakeholders to be involved with information governance, and these stakeholders should include health information management (HIM) personnel. HIM roles in the IG process might include serving as:

- Data overseers of patient data
- Auditors of financial, quality, and risk information
- Reviewers of policies and procedures for the purpose of identifying compliance gaps

HIM professionals are instrumental in helping to create (along with Information Technologists) the patient information roadmap.

## Data Analysis Tools

In the healthcare marketplace, there are many data analytical software packages available for purchase. In Excel, PivotTables are an excellent tool to summarize data into categories and filter the data in various meaningful ways. Excel also offers the option of working with frequency tables, which provide a means of summarizing data based on how often each data element occurs. Excel provides a means of displaying data in an effective manner through the use of tables and charts. In addition to Excel, healthcare data analysts can use predictive modeling to analyze historical data for the purpose of identifying patterns upon which to base future decisions. Descriptive and inferential statistics are two more types of data analysis, which can be meaningful to a healthcare organization. Types of descriptive and inferential statistics are: central tendency, mean (e.g., geometric length of stay) or average (e.g., average length of stay), median, mode, percentiles, range, standard deviation, and confidence intervals.

## Patient-Specific Documentation from Other Sources

### HIE

Health Information Exchange (HIE) refers to the electronic method of accessing and/or sharing patient health information (PHI) among healthcare providers as well as allowing patients to access their own information through secure web-based portals. The capability of electronically accessing and sharing PHI is an efficient means to improve the quality of patient care. Timely sharing of PHI improves decision making at the point of care. It also reduces the number of medication errors and eliminates duplicate testing. HIE is a key component of successful healthcare reform. It promotes the interoperability and meaningful use of health information. Through the means of HIE, healthcare costs are reduced.

### *Key Forms*

Health Information Exchange (HIE) refers to the electronic method of accessing and/or sharing patient health information (PHI) among healthcare providers as well as allowing patients to access their own information through secure web-based portals. There are three types of HIE: direct, query-based, and consumer-mediated. Direct exchange occurs between healthcare providers to coordinate care. Examples of direct exchange information that may be shared are laboratory tests results and discharge summaries. Query-based exchange occurs when providers request information, usually for unplanned episodes of care such as emergency department visit. Consumer-mediated exchange is available for patients to control the use of their PHI among providers (e.g., identifying and correcting incorrect health information).

### *Benefits*

Health Information Exchange (HIE) refers to the electronic method of accessing and/or sharing patient health information (PHI) among healthcare providers as well as allowing patients to access their own information through secure web-based portals. The many benefits to electronic HIE can include:

- Reduction in medication errors because the provider is able to see which drugs have already been prescribed or what dosages have been provided.
- Reduction in medical errors because the provider can access information quickly to obtain knowledge about diagnoses and prognosis.
- Quality of patient care improved as healthcare providers are able to administer more effective care and treatment secondary to the availability of PHI.
- Reduction in paperwork as communication between providers occurs electronically.
- Elimination of duplicate testing because providers are able to know which tests have already been completed.
- Promotes interoperability between electronic health records (EHRs) among healthcare providers.
- Reduction in healthcare costs secondary to time saved pertaining to the completion of paperwork.

## ONC for Health Information Technology

The Office of the National Coordinator for Health Information Technology (ONC) is responsible for leading the movement to promote health information exchange (HIE). HIE is growing in popularity among healthcare providers. As a result, the ONC has established a common set of guiding principles as part of the nationwide strategy to endorse HIE. The guiding principles include the:

- Establishment of clear goals for HIE
- Establishment of measures of success
- Development of policies and standards
- Identification of interoperability issues and associated costs
- Inclusion of the patient in the control of his/her health information

# Master Patient Index

## MPI

The master patient index (MPI) is a data repository of all patients who have ever been admitted or treated at a healthcare organization. The MPI is the source of truth to reference when attempting to locate patient records. The American Hospital Association (AHA) requires that certain patient information be maintained in the MPI (e.g., patient's full name, address, identifying number such as an account number and/or medical record number, and patient's birth date). Sometimes, additional information may be included such as gender, ethnicity, admission/discharge dates, and discharge disposition. Prior to the onset of the electronic health record, the MPI was managed by preparing an index card for every patient, which was maintained in an alphabetical file. The MPI in the electronic world collects the same data as the old manual systems. The electronic MPI is often created by and accessible from electronic health records, and in large healthcare systems, there will most likely be an enterprise master patient index (EMPI). An EMPI links together smaller MPIs that are contained within separate systems, such as outpatient clinics, rehab facilities, and hospitals.

## Management of Patient Identification

Accurate and consistent patient identification is an absolute necessity in today's healthcare environment, especially with an emphasis upon patient safety. Without proper patient identification, the possibilities of medication administration errors or blood transfusion administration errors can be a reality with unfortunate consequences. Therefore, a healthcare entity must have an effectively managed master patient index (MPI) or enterprise master patient index (EMPI). Some of the most common inconsistencies in MPI or EMPI platforms are duplicates and overlays. Duplicates refer to one patient with multiple medical record numbers or other patient identifiers, and overlays refer to two patient records incorporated into one medical record number. Both can cause serious adverse patient events, and, therefore, it is imperative that health information management (HIM) departments supervise the MPI/EMPI daily.

## RETENTION REQUIREMENTS FOR THE PATIENT INDEX

The master patient index (MPI) is a data repository of all patients who have ever been admitted or treated at a healthcare organization. The MPI may be manual or electronic system. For manual systems, the index cards containing the patient information may be retained in an incorruptible format, such as microfilm or microfiche, and may be kept onsite or offsite. For electronic indices, the patient information should be retained in the archived state. The recommended retention period for these indices is at least 10 years, unless state law specifies a different time frame. It is important to remember to always follow the strictest regulation. Retention time frames are influenced by federal and state laws, Medicare, and statute of limitations.

# Health Data Standards

## HEALTH DATA STANDARDS

Data standardization can be defined as the standardization of data elements (basic units of information that are unique with distinct values). Health data should be standardized in terms of defining what data to collect, deciding how the data will be represented, and knowing how it will be transmitted across various electronic systems. In order to standardize data, certain decisions will need to be determined upfront. For example: All data elements will need to be defined; data formatting will need to be implemented so that electronic transmissions can be exchanged seamlessly; and, medical and conceptual terminologies will need to be defined.

## HEALTHCARE BENCHMARKING

Healthcare benchmarking is the process of analyzing data for the purpose of identifying strengths and weaknesses and then implementing practices that lead to superior performance. Benchmarking allows a healthcare entity to compare itself against other healthcare organizations throughout the United States, and subsequently improve upon workflow processes. Of course, benchmarking is also aimed at improving coding performance, which in turn impacts revenue. Providers should be informed of benchmarking results of their associated healthcare organization. Benchmarking of coded data is an indirect reflection of providers' documentation practices. In other words, if a provider's documentation is insufficient, assigned codes and subsequent reimbursement will be adversely affected, and the benchmarking results will be noticeable in comparison to national coding results.

## EFFECTIVE TRAINING FOR PROVIDERS REGARDING HEALTH DATA, CODING, AND DOCUMENTATION STANDARDS

Effective training platforms for hospital-affiliated providers should be conducted with the understanding that providers are interested in the patient-care perspective more so than the coding classification system. Physician education sessions should be provided as continuing medical education opportunities, and the goal should be to inform the provider of how effective documentation practices will affect his/her quality outcomes and pay-for-performance initiatives. Departmental medical staff meetings or quarterly staff meetings are excellent opportunities to cover documentation improvement practices. One-on-one educational sessions tend to be the best approach because the hospital's own documentation practices can be highlighted. The intervention of a physician advisor in educational efforts is the most effective approach to improving documentation practices because the communication is peer-to-peer and better received. Coding roundtables are educational sessions that focus on coding, data analysis, and documentation improvement topics. This can be an opportunity for coders, clinical documentation improvement specialists (CDIS), and physicians to collaborate and discuss opportunities for process change.

## Interpreting Reports for Data Analysis

### COMMON REPORTS USED FOR DATA ANALYTICS

In the health information field, data analytics is a common daily task. Obtaining meaningful and relevant data is the primary objective. The following are examples of common data analytical reports generated by health information professionals:

- Calculation of readmission rates
- Case mix index analysis
- Monitoring of MCC/CC rates
- Monitoring of mortality rates
- Monitoring data dictionary statistics
- Trending inpatient and outpatient coding accuracy rates
- Trending average length of stay
- Monitoring financial impact of DRG and/or APC changes
- Monitoring adverse drug reactions
- Monitoring RAC appeals
- Monitoring payer denials

With more and more healthcare entities understanding the power of data analysis, the possibilities for additional data monitoring and trending are endless

### PIVOTTABLES AND PIVOTCHARTS IN EXCEL

In Excel, PivotTables are an excellent tool to summarize data into categories and filter the data in various meaningful ways. An HIM analyst whose responsibility may be data collection and data comparison, will find that PivotTables make data collection and comparison an easy task to complete. Once the data are categorized and filtered within a PivotTable, a PivotChart can be created for presentation purposes. To create the PivotChart, the HIM data analyst must select the data from the PivotTable, choose the best chart style (e.g., bar, column) to represent the data, and generate the chart. The PivotTable and PivotCharts can be manipulated on a prescribed time table (e.g., for quarterly reporting purposes) with the addition of new data.

### BIG DATA

Big data is referenced in this fashion for three reasons:

1. the sheer volume of data that is available,
2. the increasing frequency with which data are made available
3. the many forms of data

The volume of healthcare data has grown exponentially in the last few years, and is projected to more than triple in the upcoming years. The frequency of data through various mediums (e.g., social media, chips, monitoring devices) has increased significantly as well, all adding to the growth of available data. The many forms of data that are now available include emails, text messages, audio/video, scanned documents, etc. Big data has the potential to positively impact healthcare as it will help in understanding historical healthcare practices as well as understanding future healthcare implications.

## Components of the Medical Record

### SEMANTIC CONTENT OF AN EHR

An electronic health record (EHR) is a record of a patient's healthcare journey composed of electronic documents from various electronic systems. Prior to the EHR era, health information was maintained in paper records. Upon a patient's discharge, the paper records were retrieved from the hospital floors and assembled in a certain prescribed order in the HIM department. In today's EHR environment, assembly of the information means that it should be available in a logical and meaningful manner for the healthcare employee's use. Therefore, uniformity and standardization of data collection points (or fields) should be the norm. In an EHR environment, semantic content, or the inherent meaning of each data element, must retain its meaning throughout its lifetime as this promotes data integrity.

### BRINGING ALL INFORMATION TOGETHER TO GENERATE AN ELECTRONIC RECORD

An electronic record (EHR) is "assembled" through different means of capture: scanned paper documents, automatic feeds, and manual entry. Scanned paper documents or document imaging processes are necessary for paper documents to become a part of the EHR. Primarily, this process involves three steps: document preparation (e.g., removing staples, repairing tears, and organizing papers by document type), document scanning (e.g., actual physical scanning and conversion to an electronic image), and document quality control and indexing (e.g., HIM personnel check each individual image for quality and index the image based on document type). Automatic feeds of certain reports also become part of an EHR, such as the admissions/discharges/transfer (ADT) transaction report, transcribed reports, and radiology reports. Manual entry of data by clinicians into predefined templates of the EHR is also a means of data capture. Once these steps are completed, each account is processed through coding and deficiency management and finally physician authentication.

### COMPONENTS OF A MEDICAL RECORD

Although there are no requirements for what should be included in a medical record, there are several components that are recommended in order for a record to be considered complete. The first component is a personal identification number that, when used, is automatically generated by an electronic health record system when the patient schedules their first appointment. It serves to distinguish a patient from other patients who may have a similar name or the same name. A medical record should also contain a full history of the patient. This includes past medical history (i.e., chronic conditions, pregnancies), surgical history, family history (i.e., cause of death of immediate family members), and social history (i.e., nicotine or alcohol use). Other miscellaneous information to be included are demographics, immunizations, drug allergies, and medical directives.

### PHYSICIAN'S CLINICAL NOTES

What a physician documents in their clinical notes often has a direct impact on the continuity and quality of care provided to a patient, especially when multiple physicians are involved. Additionally, an insurance company can choose to deny or recoup payment for services that are rendered but not properly documented by a physician. Therefore, a well-documented clinical note should include the date and reason for the current visit, pertinent positive and negative exam findings, a diagnosis of the patient's condition and preexisting comorbidities, a treatment plan or recommendation, medications newly prescribed or renewed, educational information relayed to the patient, and a recommended follow-up date.

# Compliance

## Documentation

### CODING COMPLIANCE
Coding compliance is an important function of healthcare operations secondary to federal regulations. Code assignments must be supported by clinical documentation in order to avoid denials by payers and/or appeal their decisions. Discrepancies between coded data and supporting documentation can be identified through data analytics and/or through internal auditing processes. Through the auditing of records identified as high-risk accounts (based on diagnosis-related groups), internal auditors identify documentation insufficiencies/discrepancies. For example, a coder assigns the principal diagnosis as lung mass. However, upon closer inspection of the medical record documentation, the internal auditor finds documentation of lung carcinoma with metastases to the mediastinal lymph nodes. Both diagnoses have corresponding codes that the coder missed entirely, and both diagnoses and their corresponding codes correlate to a positive financial impact.

### MEASURING CODING COMPLIANCE EFFECTIVENESS WITHIN A HEALTHCARE ORGANIZATION
Coding compliance is an important function of healthcare operations secondary to federal regulations. Code assignments must be supported by clinical documentation in order to avoid denials by payers and/or appeal their decisions. Discrepancies between coded data and supporting documentation can be identified through data analytics and/or through internal auditing processes. Through the auditing of records identified as high-risk accounts (based on diagnosis-related groups), internal auditors identify documentation insufficiencies/discrepancies. For example, a coder assigns the principal diagnosis as lung mass. However, upon closer inspection of the medical record documentation, the internal auditor finds documentation of lung carcinoma with metastases to the mediastinal lymph nodes. Both diagnoses have corresponding codes which the coder missed entirely, and both diagnoses and their corresponding codes correlate to a positive financial impact.

### DETERMINING WHICH DOCUMENTED TERMS MATCH THE ICD-10-PCS CODE DESCRIPTIONS
With the implementation of ICD-10-PCS coding conventions came many new procedural terms used to construct the PCS codes. Physicians are not responsible for using the exact terminology related to the root operation. Rather, it is the coder's responsibility to comprehend the physician's documentation and equate the terminology to the correct PCS root operation. Additionally, a coder should not query a physician when his/her documentation is clear as to which PCS root operational term is applicable. For example, if a physician documents "total mastectomy," the coder should know that the root operation is "resection" because the PCS definition of resection is "cutting off, without replacement, *all* of a body part."

### CONFLICTING DOCUMENTATION PROCESS
Some patients admitted to an inpatient status in the hospital will be assessed by multiple physicians. Inevitably, the documentation of the various physicians will conflict. For example, the attending physician may document acute renal "failure," but the nephrology consultant documents acute renal "disease." Since failure and disease in this particular case equate to different codes, the coder will need clarification, and that clarification is best achieved through the initiation of a query. The query would need to reveal the conflicting information and ask for the final decision as to which diagnosis is correct. Other clinical indicators should be a part of the query in order to demonstrate to the physician why the information is conflicting. For example, in this acute renal

failure versus disease scenario, the coder may choose to include the clinical indicators pertaining to a rise in the BUN/creatinine as well as the urine output amounts.

# Ethical Coding

## AHIMA's Standards of Ethical Coding

The American Health Information Management Association (AHIMA) has issued standards pertaining to ethical coding. The standards reflect the expectations for professional coding conduct in diagnostic and procedural coding as well as abstracting of health information. The standards are available for reference on AHIMA's website, but an abbreviated version follows:

- Accurate, complete, and consistent coding practices are required.
- Coding compliance with regulatory guidelines is expected regarding reimbursement and data reporting.
- Documentation must support assigned codes.
- Provider queries are acceptable for the purpose of documentation clarification.
- Code assignments must not be misrepresented.
- Inappropriate assignment of codes for financial gain is prohibited.
- Continuing education to advance coding knowledge is necessary.
- Maintain confidentiality of patient health information.

## Ensuring Ethical Coding

Certified coders and/or clinical documentation improvement specialist (CDIS) are obligated to follow the ethical standards published by the American Health Information Management Association (AHIMA). Many healthcare organizations implement steps to ensure the ethical coding standards are followed by their coding and/or CDIS employees. These steps may include any of the following:

- Requirement of coding/CDIS employees to acknowledge a code of conduct.
- Implementation of policies and procedures that address ethical coding standards.
- Issuance of compliance alerts and/or advisory memos by regulatory compliance departments to frequently remind employees of corporate expectations/requirements.
- Implementation of annual education webinars that address ethical coding standards.

# Physician Queries

## Initiating a Physician Query

Initiation of a physician query is appropriate when documentation within the medical record fails to provide the necessary information needed by the coder to make an informed decision about a code assignment. Issues such as legibility, completeness, clarity, or consistency may be what prompts the initiation of a query. The query may be done either concurrently by a clinical documentation information specialist (CDIS) or retrospectively by a coder. Physician queries must be phrased in such a way that it does not appear that the CDIS or coder is leading the physician to a certain diagnosis. Physician queries must also provide clinical indicators from the existing documentation that explains the CDIS's or coder's reasoning to the queried physician.

There are several reasons why a coder would initiate a physician's query. If a diagnosis and/or procedure has been determined to meet the American Hospital Association's (AHA's) ICD-10 Official Coding Guidelines for reporting but the diagnosis and/or procedure has not been clearly stated within the documentation, then a query may be necessary. Reasons why initiation of a query may occur would be: 1) when a present on admission (POA) indicator is not clearly stated and the coder must know this information in order to meet the federal requirement to report POA status, or 2) when conflicting, ambiguous, or incomplete documentation is present. Query templates may be a helpful tool for coders to use when initiating queries since they promote query standardization.

## INTENT OF A PHYSICIAN QUERY

A physician query is a tool of communication between CDISs/Coders and physicians to clarify incomplete, ambiguous, or conflicting documentation in the medical record. The intention of the communication tool is to facilitate completeness, accuracy, consistency, and timely documentation for coding and reporting practices. Queries are an essential tool that provides additional clarification that allows coding and reporting to the highest level of specificity. It is best for the physician's query to be maintained as a permanent part of the medical record since it is considered to be supporting documentation for assigned codes.

## REQUIRED COMPONENTS OF A QUERY

A physician query should include certain components in order to be a valid and/or compliant query. These components should be:

- Name of the contact individual submitting the query
- Patient's date of service (DOS)
- Patient's name
- Medical Record Number
- Account Number
- Date of the query
- Name of the MD being queried
- Clinical indicators pertinent to the condition/diagnosis/procedure in question
- Statement of the issue in the form of a question

Examples of when queries may be issued are:

- Determine if a diagnosis was present on admission (POA)
- Clarify what specific organism was the cause and effect of an infectious disease
- Clarify the severity of asthma
- Clarify the particular stage of chronic kidney disease (CKD)
- Clarify if a diagnosis was ruled in or ruled out
- Determine which diagnosis or procedure is applicable when conflicting information exists
- Clarify whether or not pneumonia was caused by aspiration

## CLINICAL INDICATORS

Compliant coding is dependent on the accuracy and completeness of documentation. In some cases, healthcare documentation is not sufficient to support code assignments, and in those cases, physician queries are necessary. Queries must contain certain elements, and clinical indicators are one of the elements. Clinical indicators refer to clinical clues, such as elevated temperature, abnormal vital signs, elevated white blood cell count levels, etc., which could indicate or support certain diagnoses. For example, if a provider fails to document the diagnosis of sepsis, but there are clinical indicators that point to its diagnosis, a query might be warranted. The coder or clinical documentation improvement specialist (CDIS) might include the following clinical indicators in the query: temperature 103°F, WBC 18,500, blood pressure 70/40 (hypotension). These three clinical clues might indicate the diagnosis of sepsis, and the physician would consider these indicators to make a decision.

## Leading Query

A leading query can be defined as one that is not supported by the clinical elements contained within the medical record, or it can be defined as a query that directs a healthcare provider to a specific diagnosis or procedure. Leading a provider to a specific diagnosis or procedure is an unbalanced approach because it appears to prompt the provider to make only one decision. A coder or clinical documentation improvement specialist (CDIS) should never suggest only one diagnostic or procedural option because coders/CDIS are not credentialed healthcare providers.

Leading provider/physician queries are not acceptable in healthcare. The following are examples of inappropriate leading queries:

- A query that provides the physician with options that only lead to additional reimbursement.
- A query that does not contain all the required clinical indicators that paint the full clinical picture of the patient's condition.
- A query wherein the statements are directive in nature, such as indicating what the provider should document, rather than querying the provider for his/her professional determination of the clinical facts.
- A query that leads the provider to one desired outcome.
- A query that omits reasonable clinically supported options.
- A query that omits an option that no additional documentation or clarification may be provided.

## Standardized Physician Query Forms

The use of standardized physician query forms by coders and/or clinical documentation improvement specialists (CDIS) is an efficient way to obtain compliant queries. Standardized queries should be created based on disease processes or circumstances that are most likely to require a query (e.g., sepsis, acuity of respiratory failure, specificity of renal failure, whether a diagnosis was ruled in or ruled out). Through the utilization of standardized forms with specified clinical indicators, three objectives should be accomplished: 1) overall documentation improvement should be noted, 2) potential coding errors due to poor documentation practices should be avoided, and 3) potential compliance issues related to leading queries should be mitigated.

## Query Formatting

There are several ways to generate a query. Compliant query forms will allow for open-ended questions, multiple choice query formats, and/or limited yes/no query formats. An example of open-ended query might appear in this format: "Based upon your clinical judgment, please provide a diagnosis that represents the following clinical indicators: temperature 102°F, cellulitis around ankle with open wound, white blood cell count 15,000." An example of a multiple choice query might appear in this format: "Per the Discharge Summary, the patient has congestive heart failure (CHF). Can the CHF be further specified as: 1) acute systolic CHF, 2) acute on chronic systolic CHF, 3) acute diastolic CHF, 4) acute on chronic diastolic CHF, or 5) undetermined?" An example of a yes/no query might appear in this format: "Was the sepsis documented in the Discharge Summary present on admission? Yes, No, clinically unable to determine."

# Coding Changes

## ANNUAL CODING CHANGES THAT OCCUR FOR BOTH ICD-10 AND CPT

Coding changes are implemented annually for both ICD-10-CM/PCS and CPT. The updates are implemented at different times during the year. ICD-10-CM/PCS changes are implemented on October 1, 20xx, and CPT coding updates are implemented on January 1, 20xx. The ICD-10-CM updates for 2017 have been released by CMS and are rather significant with 1,974 additions, 311 deletions, and 425 revisions. The ICD-10-PCS updates for 2017 include 3,827 additions, 491 revisions, and 12 deletions. CPT coding updates will also include additions, deletions, and revisions. Updates are made available to healthcare entities through online webinars and/or coding workshops.

## IMPORTANT CODING CHANGES RESOURCES

An experienced coder understands the importance of accessing reliable resources for compliant coding. Coding Clinic, CPT Assistant, and 3M Nosology are reliable resources frequently referenced by seasoned coders. The American Hospital Association (AHA) publishes the Coding Clinic, an official publication of coding guidelines and advice. The AHA Central Office works with the National Center for Health Statistics (NCHS) and CMS to maintain the integrity of the ICD-10 coding classification system. CPT Assistant is published and maintained by the American Medical Association (AMA) as the official word on proper CPT coding. 3M Nosology is a support system whose employees field coding questions and provide advice on appropriate code assignment. All three resources are valuable tools for coding professionals.

## TIMING OF CODING UPDATES FOR ICD-10 AND FOR CPT

Coding changes are implemented annually for both ICD-10-CM/PCS and CPT. The updates are implemented at different times during the year. ICD-10-CM/PCS changes are implemented on October 1, 20xx, and CPT coding updates are implemented on January 1, 20xx. CMS, the Centers for Disease Control (CDC), and the National Center for Health Statistics (NCHS) collaborate through a federal committee known as the ICD-10 Coordination and Maintenance Committee for the purpose of ICD-10 code update implementation. The CPT Editorial Panel, authorized by the American Medical Association (AMA), and the CPT Advisory Committee are responsible for CPT annual updates.

## ICD-10 CODING CHANGES THAT OCCURRED ON OCTOBER 1, 2015

October 1, 2015 is the date well known to health information management (HIM) professionals. It was the much anticipated time when the ninth edition of the International Classification of Diseases (ICD) was finally retired, and the ICD-10 coding system was implemented. The ninth edition had been in effect for 30 years, and with the exponential growth in healthcare technology, ICD-9 lacked sufficient detail. Therefore, CMS mandated the change for any healthcare provider covered by the Health Insurance Portability and Accountability Act (HIPAA). Effective on October 1, 2015, any healthcare provider who had been submitting ICD-9 codes on claims were now required to switch to ICD-10.

## EQUIVALENCE MAPPINGS

General equivalence mappings (GEMs) demonstrate a network of relationships between ICD-9 codes and ICD-10 codes. It is a bidirectional map. GEMs are a translation reference tool; they may be referred to as crosswalks. There are approximately 250,000 GEMs. GEMs were created due to the complexity of structural changes between the two code sets. The purpose of GEMs is to assist coders in finding a corresponding procedural code if there is no obvious correlation. It is important for a coder to know that GEMs should never replace the utilization of the ICD-9 or ICD-10. Up-to-date GEMs are available for review on the CMS website.

## Mapping Pathways

Through the utilization of a code map, one is able to either forward map or backward map. Forward mapping is when the ICD-9 code is available and an ICD-10 code is needed, and backward mapping is the opposite—an ICD-10 code is available, but an ICD-9 code is needed. It is important to understand that GEMs do not necessarily have a 1:1 match between the two code sets. For example, it is estimated that less than 25% of ICD-9 codes can be mapped to an ICD-10 code. Obviously, there are ICD-9 codes that map to multiple ICD-10 codes, and this is known as one-to-many mapping, and in these cases, the multiple ICD-10 codes are more specific than the ICD-9 codes. Since there is a GEM concept for one-to-many mapping, it is also important to understand that there is a many-to-one mapping. In these cases, more than one ICD-9 code is required to provide a match to a single ICD-10 code.

## How a Code Becomes a Code

A diagnosis and/or procedure is assigned its own code after going through a process of consideration by an advisory healthcare panel. The advisory panel, whether considering ICD-10 codes or CPT classification codes, will collaborate multiple times throughout the year to solicit advice from physicians, surgeons, medical device manufacturers, developers of diagnostic tests, and other advisors from various healthcare arenas. Applications for code additions and changes may be submitted by healthcare entities to the advisory panel, and the outcome may be the addition of a new code, referral to a work group for further study, postponement to a future meeting, or rejection of the request.

## Updating a Charge Ticket

### Physician's Office

In order to prevent payer denials, a physician's office should update a charge ticket or encounter form annually (at a minimum) or as significant coding/charging changes occur. By proactively making the necessary changes to a charge ticket, denials on the back end are reduced or avoided. Therefore, it is best to review ICD-10 and CPT codes as they are updated annually to ensure the ticket includes the updates. Code descriptions on the charge ticket should also be assessed to ensure that the terminology is correct and not misleading to a health professional who might "check the wrong box" based upon the code title rather than the actual code.

### Hospital

In order to prevent payer denials, a hospital should update departmental charge tickets annually (at a minimum) or as significant coding/charging changes occur. The same changes should also be coordinated with the hospital chargemaster. By proactively making the necessary changes to a charge ticket and the chargemaster, denials on the back end are reduced or avoided. Therefore, it is best to review ICD-10 and CPT codes as they are updated annually to ensure the departmental tickets and chargemaster include the updates. Code descriptions should also be assessed to ensure that the terminology is correct and not misleading to a health professional who might select the wrong code/charge based on an incorrect title.

### Chargemaster

A hospital has a database that contains all charges for services rendered. This database is known as the chargemaster or charge description master (CDM). The CDM is the core of a hospital's revenue cycle. Each hospital department is responsible for entering the type of service or supply provided to a patient. Each procedure, supply, or service has its own unique item number. For each charge, a

CPT/HCPCS code and revenue code as well as other financial elements are assigned. The functions of the CDM are to not only assign charges, but also to produce itemized statements, produce a valid claim, monitor costs, and generate financial reporting.

A hospital's chargemaster is composed of certain key elements. The typical data elements could be the following:

- Charge description: Each charge has a title that describes the charge whether it is a supply, a medication, a procedure, etc.
- CPT/HCPCS code and modifiers: A CPT or HCPCS code may be assigned to a specific procedure or supply, and applicable modifiers may be built in to the charge as well. Of note, not all charges will have a corresponding CPT/HCPCS code or modifier.
- Revenue code: This is a three-digit number that represents the location of the patient when the service was rendered or the type of service the patient received.
- Charge dollar amount: This is the cost associated with the service or supply provided.
- Charge code: This is the unique number assigned to each item listed in the Chargemaster. It is also known as the CDM number.
- Charge status: This represents whether or not the charge has been allocated to the patient's account and its payment or denial status.

## Educating Providers on Compliant Coding

### PHYSICIAN CHAMPIONS IN CODING COMPLIANCE

Accurate and compliant coding is dependent upon complete and detailed documentation by the healthcare provider. The challenge for HIM professionals is convincing physicians of the importance of their role in providing valuable supportive documentation. Therefore, physician champions should be engaged in the process. Advice regarding effective documentation practices is better received by physicians from physician champions. Physician champions can also stress to other physicians how efficient supportive documentation impacts the provider's own quality measures in addition to the hospital's quality measures.

### PHYSICIAN DOCUMENTATION VULNERABILITIES

Physician/Provider documentation always has room for improvement, especially in a world of constantly changing healthcare regulations. The Office of Inspector General (OIG) is well aware of documentation vulnerabilities and publish these annually in their OIG Work Plan. Some of the targeted areas for review of documentation are: cloned notes, diagnosis specificity, and medical necessity. Cloned notes refer to previously documented notes that have been copied and pasted. A cloned note can provide inaccurate information for the current visit, which can adversely impact patient care. The vulnerability behind diagnosis specificity centers on missed opportunities for the identification of laterality, disease manifestation, anatomical location, etc. A final vulnerability exists in terms of medical necessity, which may not be supported with appropriate documentation, and subsequent payer denials occur.

### HEALTHCARE PROVIDERS MUST NOW BE MORE SPECIFIC WITH DOCUMENTATION PRACTICES

With the implementation of ICD-10 coding classification system, the expectation for more in-depth documentation became a reality. ICD-10 brought about major changes in the areas of: classification axes, laterality, obstetrical trimester specificity, expansion of certain codes, and complications. ICD-10 is a multiaxial system with the primary axis of anatomy. Many diseases, however, are organized in ICD-10 based upon several axes such as etiology, site, or morphology. Laterality also demands more specific documentation as many conditions (e.g., fractures, burns, ulcers) must now be identified by the affected side of the body in order to assign an accurate ICD-10 code. For any complications that arise during a pregnancy, obstetrical coding now requires the time frame of the complication (e.g., trimester). Code expansion in terms of diagnoses related to alcohol and drugs requires more specific documentation. ICD-10 codes for complications that arise postoperatively have been expanded, requiring more specific documentation. All of these changes necessitate improved documentation by healthcare providers.

## External Audits

### HEALTHCARE COMPLIANCE AUDIT

Multiple types of healthcare compliance audits are being conducted in the present age. To understand the purpose of a compliance audit, one must understand the different types of audits. Hospitals should be prepared in the following areas (at a minimum) where audits are likely to occur: HIPAA, meaningful use, provider-based status, outlier payments, Medicare's Two-Midnight Rule, inpatient claims for mechanical ventilation, ambulatory surgery centers payment system, anesthesia services, outpatient rehab services, immunosuppressive drug claims, hospice and home health services, etc. The list of potential audits by external agencies is extensive. The Office of Inspector General (OIG) publishes a Work Plan for each fiscal year, and this plan is an excellent indicator of where hospitals, skilled nursing facilities, pharmacies, clinics, etc., should focus their attention for internal auditing. The purpose behind each of these external auditors essentially is to identify fraud, waste, and abuse. They are also looking for opportunities to improve healthcare efficiency, and in many cases, this includes holding accountable those who violate federal healthcare laws.

### GOVERNMENTAL AUDITS

Federal auditors have the authority to review Medicare and Medicaid claims submitted by providers. Some of federal government audit entities are Medicare Recovery Audit Contractor (RAC), Office of Inspector General (OIG), Zone Program Integrity Contractor (ZPIC), and Department of Justice (DOJ). Depending upon the entity involved, the auditor will have different scopes of work, and the number of accounts reviewed, timeline of the audit, and appeals process will vary among the auditors. The RAC's goal is to reduce Medicare improper payments. The focus of the OIG, DOJ, and ZPICs is on fraud and abuse. Therefore, it is imperative that healthcare organizations be prepared for governmental audits.

### EXTERNAL AUDITS THAT MAY BE REQUESTED OF A HOSPITAL

Hospitals experience audits from external agencies on a regular basis. The external auditors may be representatives of various federal agencies (e.g., Office of Inspector General, Department of Justice, Medicare Administrative Contractors). They may also represent commercial insurers (e.g., Blue Cross/Blue Shield). The types of audits requested may pertain to charges (e.g., pharmaceutical, supplies), coding, medical necessity, fraud, etc. Complete documentation is key to proving to the external auditor that a submitted claim is valid and meets regulatory compliance.

### PREPARING FOR EXTERNAL AUDITS

Hospitals experience audits from external agencies on a regular basis. The external auditors may be representatives of various federal agencies (e.g., Office of Inspector General, Department of Justice, Medicare Administrative Contractors). They may also represent commercial insurers (e.g., Blue Cross/Blue Shield). The types of audits requested may pertain to charges (e.g., pharmaceutical, supplies), coding, medical necessity, fraud, contracts, policies, etc. Preparation should include the development and implementation of policies and procedures, organizational education regarding each department's responsibility during an audit, identification of individuals internally who should be involved in the audits, and determination of appeals processes.

## EMTALA Audit

EMTALA is the acronym for Emergency Medical Treatment and Labor Act. Congress enacted EMTALA in 1986 to ensure that all people would have access to emergency services regardless of the individual's ability to pay. This law mandates hospitals to provide stabilizing treatment for a patient with an emergency medical condition, and if unable to stabilize the patient, the hospital is required to transfer the patient to a facility where stabilization can occur. EMTALA is enforced by CMS as well as the Office of Inspector General (OIG), and either entity may conduct an audit. To prepare for an EMTALA audit, hospitals should review their EMTALA and transfer policies and procedures (P&Ps), medical staff bylaws, physician on-call lists, emergency workflows, emergency department transfer form, and emergency department signage. P&Ps should be up-to-date with EMTALA guidance. Medical staff bylaws should indicate who is allowed to perform the medical screening exam. The emergency workflow should be EMTALA compliant, and signage should be easy to understand and follow from the patient's perspective. The transfer forms must be completed in their entirety, and on-call lists must correspond with documentation in the medical record.

# Information Technologies

## Navigating Throughout the EHR

### ELECTRONIC HEALTH RECORD

An electronic health record (EHR) is a digital version of patients' health information. EHRs provide the means to access patients' health information instantly and for more than one user at a time across multiple healthcare venues. While EHRs do contain the same health information found in patients' paper records (e.g., administrative and billing data, demographics, medical history, physical examination, diagnoses, procedures, medications, laboratory values, radiology tests), an EHR is a more valuable tool to the healthcare provider than a paper record because the capability exists to streamline efficient workflow processes in an automated environment. Additionally, the capability exists to capture more relevant data than one would be able to collect from a paper chart.

Use of an electronic health record (EHR) boasts many benefits. One of the most obvious benefits is the fact that any patient's health information may be accessed instantly by more than one user across innumerable organizations. In other words, it is available whenever and wherever it is needed by whomever (healthcare practitioner) needs it. Because of the ease of access, patient care is improved whether it is advantageous to the provider (e.g., enhanced decision support, legible documentation), or advantageous to the patient (e.g., convenience of e-prescriptions, patient portal access). Coordination of care between providers is also improved, and cost and time savings related to EHR use are beneficial.

The healthcare information contained within an electronic health record (EHR) is similar to the information housed in a paper health record. Administrative and billing data, demographics, medical history, physical examination, diagnoses, procedures, medications, laboratory values, radiology tests, etc., are found in both versions. The advantages of an EHR are numerous. It can automatically identify contraindications between medications and/or allergies and alert the provider to a potential adverse event. EHRs can also alert a provider in an emergency situation of life-threatening allergies. This is especially important with an unconscious patient who is unable to verbalize known allergies. EHRs can also prevent duplication of tests, thus promoting cost savings. This is just a sampling of types of information contained within an EHR; the list is extensive.

### *HIM ROLES AND RESPONSIBILITIES*

Health Information Management (HIM) professionals are key to the successful adoption of an electronic health record (EHR). In fact, an HIM professional must be in a leadership position when it comes to ensuring that the EHR is legally compliant. The HIM professional would be instrumental in developing policies and procedures pertaining to the creation and maintenance of the legal record. Training/Education of EHR navigation would also be a key responsibility for an HIM leader to the healthcare entity. These individuals are trained to ensure privacy, quality, and integrity of health information. Data analytics and the development of decision-support systems would also be a primary responsibility of an HIM professional.

### *USING TEMPLATES AND PROMPTS*

Templates and prompts are tools used in the development of electronic health records (EHRs). They differ in their purpose with templates used to collect, present, and organize data elements, and prompts used to remind providers of required documentation. The use of templates and prompts requires diligent planning and subsequent maintenance in order to make any necessary

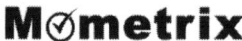

changes. Templates are beneficial as they promote standardization, streamlined workflow processes, time savings, increased timely chart completion, consistent data capture, etc. Prompts are beneficial as they promote documentation compliance with regulatory requirements.

## Encoding and Grouping Software

### ENCODER

An encoder is an electronic tool that receives diagnostic or procedural data manually entered by a coder, and then converts the data into a numerical code. An encoder is a logic-driven tool that prompts the coder through several choices/options until the appropriate code is achieved. This tool promotes consistency and accuracy because it potentially prevents the coder from missing a key piece of information. In many computer-assisted coding (CAC) programs, the encoder is an integral part. The encoder serves the same purpose in CAC as it does in a stand-alone encoder—logically guide the coder to the appropriate code selection based upon the providers' documentation. Whether a coder uses a stand-alone encoder, a CAC encoder, or codes with an ICD-10 book only, the critical skill for the coder is to accurately and thoroughly search the health information for the diagnoses and procedures that affect the hospital stay.

An encoder is an electronic tool that receives diagnostic or procedural data manually entered by a coder, and then converts the data into a numerical code. An encoder is a logic-driven tool that prompts the coder through several choices/options until the appropriate code is achieved. Inevitably, the coder will encounter insufficient documentation that leaves the coder questioning which code to assign. In these situations, the coder should access coding references to guide in his/her code selection process. These coding references are available in an encoder. The references may include the ICD-9 and ICD-10 Official Coding Guidelines, American Hospital Association's Coding Clinics dating back to the 1990s, American Medical Association's CPT Assistant, Faye Brown's Coding Handbook, Approved Medical Abbreviation Lists, Elsevier's Anatomy Plates, etc.

## Practice Management and HIM System

### EHR SYSTEM FOR A PHYSICIAN'S PRACTICE

Many physician offices are migrating away from paper record systems to EHRs. Multiple EHR systems are available for purchase in today's market, so it is imperative that physician offices designate a work team and a strategic plan to select the best system. When considering an EHR system for a physician's practice, several elements are key to a successful choice and subsequent implementation. An efficient EHR system should promote improved patient safety, efficient delivery of health care, and effective management of acute and chronic conditions. This type of system should incorporate the obvious core functionalities related to health data, test results, order entry, decision support, communication, and reporting.

### TOP-RANKED PRACTICE MANAGEMENT SYSTEM

A practice management system is the software that runs the business side of a healthcare practice. It is usually separate from the electronic health record (EHR), which is the world where physicians primarily operate. The practice management system is the responsibility of the practice manager or the information technology (IT) department. A top-ranked practice management system in health care should include the following key components:

- An automated task management system that instructs staff on which actions to take next.
- Ability to track financial trends and improve accounts receivable workflows.

- Schedule management feature that allows calendar control of multiple providers' schedules as well as establishing rules for recurring appointments.
- Ability to submit claims electronically.
- Ability to interface with clearinghouses.
- Ability to track claim status.
- A comprehensive master patient index (MPI).
- Identification of duplicate registrations.
- Ability to track payment activity as well as collection of overdue balances.
- Evaluation of coding trends.
- Ability to stay up-to-date with changing compliance regulations.
- Simplified and streamlined workflows.

## Computer Assisted Coding Software

### CAC

Computer-assisted coding (CAC) software is a helpful aid to coders because it analyzes electronic health information for specific medical terms and phrases that correlate to numerical codes. CAC software uses natural language processing (NLP) to identify the terminology. CAC offers many benefits to a coder, such as efficiency in coding, increased production, decrease in average coding turn-around time, consistency in following coding guidelines, and decreased coding error rates. Even though coding errors rates may decrease, it is still imperative for a coder to double-check the CAC-assigned codes because CAC is capable of selecting incorrect terminology. For example, CAC may select cancer as a diagnosis to code, but in reality, the appropriate code should reflect *history of cancer*.

The daily workflow a coder might encounter using computer-assisted coding could proceed as follows:

- Coder logs into the CAC system.
- Coder selects account to code from the coding queue.
- CAC opens the electronic patient record for viewing through pre-established interfaces between CAC and the healthcare's electronic health record (EHR).
- Coder reviews the patient information and clicks on hyperlinks to review suggested codes.
- Coder is responsible for selecting the correct codes suggested by CAC.

CAC also provides hyperlinks to coding resources as a useful tool for the coder to access.

#### NATURAL LANGUAGE PROCESSING

Natural Language Processing (NLP) is an integral and important part of computer-assisted coding. NLP technology has the capability to process text as well as data fields containing text into suggested ICD-10 codes. NLP technologies differ in how they decipher narrative texts, how they recognize coding-related data, and how they integrate data between systems. An efficient CAC system will be one that correctly suggests accurate codes based on coding and/or regulatory guidelines, and through the CAC's accuracy, the coder's job is more easily accomplished. In other words, if a CAC-recommended code has supporting documentation and is an accurate recommendation, the coder can review the suggested code and documentation more quickly, thus increasing production. The best CAC system will operate with an NLP with excellent encoder functionality so that the coder does not have to access various systems of an encoder, coding references, EHR, etc.

CAC software and systems can be excellent tools in the selection of accurate diagnostic and procedural codes supported by compliant documentation. However, CAC is not without its problems. CAC does not have the capability to decipher between a present diagnosis and a history of a diagnosis. For example, a patient may have a history of colon cancer, but CAC fails to recognize the "history of" part of the phrase and instead selects colon cancer as a current illness. CAC also may select incorrect diagnoses entirely. For example, it may translate the medical abbreviation ARF for acute renal failure to acute respiratory failure incorrectly. These two examples illustrate the reasons why CAC is not 100% reliable and must require the involvement of a coder in the process.

## Auditing Code Assignments

Healthcare entities should never assume that CAC systems are 100% accurate. Therefore, it is imperative to implement a coding compliance program in which auditors review accounts on a daily basis. The volume of coded charts will far outweigh the number of auditors available to review; therefore, appropriate data analysis and filtering methods should be implemented to identify high-risk accounts. Once automated auditing tools identify the high-risk accounts, a systematic approach of auditing for compliant coding practices should occur. Any coding discrepancies should be conveyed to the coder for corrections and/or further discussion. After recommended corrections are made, rebills of corrected claims to the appropriate payer should occur.

## Pre-Bill vs. Retrospective Coding Audits

A pre-bill coding audit is an audit that is conducted before the initial claim is ever submitted to the payer. The benefit to conducting a pre-bill audit is that errors are identified and corrected proactively, which prevents payment denials and/or payment take-backs by the payer. A pre-bill audit also provides an opportunity for the auditor to identify any "red flags" which alert governmental payers of potential errors through their data analysis software. Pre-bill audits result in high reimbursement for providers because repetitive paybacks are reduced or eliminated. On the contrary, a retrospective coding audit is performed after the initial claim has been submitted to the payer, and if errors are identified during the audit, a subsequent bill with corrected errors is submitted. This results in extra work effort for the billing department and can raise red flags with payers.

## Potential Problems with CAC-Assigned Codes

Computer-assisted coding software does not diminish the role of a coder. Rather, the value of having the coder's knowledge and skills applied to the CAC process enhances the overall coding accuracy. In other words, coders will not be replaced by a machine because problems do exist with CAC. One potential problem with CAC-assigned codes pertains to the software's inability to logically decipher complicated cases, and therefore it is necessary for a coder to comprehend the coding rules correctly and assign the appropriate code(s). Another known CAC-related problem is with the software's inability to decipher current illnesses versus historical illnesses as well as illnesses related to family diseases versus personal history.

# Confidentiality & Privacy

## Ensuring Patient Confidentiality

### PATIENT CONFIDENTIALITY

Confidentiality is a core responsibility of a healthcare organization. This ethical practice requires healthcare workers (regardless of role) to keep all patients' health information private. The basic premise behind confidentiality is trust. Trust is necessary in order for the physician-patient relationship to stay intact so that sensitive information will be shared. When a patient understands their information will be kept private, he/she will be encouraged to seek out care and be open during the visit about his/her health condition. This is especially important with information pertaining to diseases of psychiatric, sexual, or drug/alcohol origins.

### PHI

Protected health information (PHI) is defined by the US Department of Health and Human Services (HHS) and is included in the Code of Federal Regulations (CFR). PHI is governed by the Health Insurance Portability and Accountability Act (HIPAA). HHS, CFR, and HIPAA support the concept that PHI data are available in electronic, paper, and/or verbal media. Electronic collection of PHI data may be created and maintained in personal computers, USB storage devices, DVDs, PDAs, etc. PHI is created or received by healthcare providers, patients, insurance payers, etc. Health information data that is individually identifiable is the data to be protected. Individual identifiers may be any of the following: patient name, address, phone number, social security number, email address.

### HIPAA

HIPAA is the acronym for Health Insurance and Portability and Accountability Act, also known as the Privacy Rule. This Act was endorsed by Congress in 2003. The Privacy Rule allows patients to have control of their own health information, all while ensuring that patients' healthcare treatment is not hindered. HIPAA defines boundaries for the use of health information and the appropriate methods to follow for disclosures. Of note, PHI may be shared between healthcare providers without obtaining a disclosure from the patient. HIPAA does enforce accountability for protecting health information, and, if violated, criminal and civil penalties do exist.

Under the HIPAA Privacy Rule, patients have rights. When patients receive healthcare services, HIPAA requires that they receive a notice of their privacy rights. This notice must describe how the healthcare entity will use/share the protected health information (PHI), and how otherwise it will not be released without appropriate consent by the patient. HIPAA also addresses patients' rights to access their own records and obtain a copy of their records, as well as the right to request an amendment to their health information, the right to request special privacy protection, and the right to access a minor's health information by a parent or legal guardian. Violations of patients' privacy rights may result in criminal or civil penalties.

### BREACH OF CONFIDENTIALITY

A healthcare privacy breach or breach of confidentiality is an inappropriate or impermissible use or disclosure of health information. This type of breach is a direct violation of Health Insurance and Portability and Accountability Act (HIPAA), also known as the Privacy Rule. A breach may occur when the security or privacy of the protected health information (PHI) is compromised. If the covered entity, responsible for the breach, can demonstrate that the PHI was not viewed or that the entity has taken steps to mitigate the risk, the release may not be considered a breach. There are other exceptions to the definition of breach, which may be described as:

- an unintentional acquisition made in good faith
- an inadvertent disclosure between healthcare entities
- a situation wherein the recipient of the PHI did not retain the information

## Enforcing Privacy and Security Rules

The Office for Civil Rights (OCR) is the governmental body responsible for the enforcement of the Privacy Rule. The OCR works in conjunction with the Department of Justice (DOJ) to investigate possible criminal cases of healthcare privacy breaches. The OCR investigates complaints of privacy breaches. They also routinely conduct reviews of healthcare entities to determine whether they are in compliance with policies pertaining to privacy. The OCR may resolve complaints of potential privacy breaches by either determining there is no violation or determining a violation did occur, which requires corrective action.

## Physician-Patient Confidentiality

The physician-patient relationship is considered to be a contractual agreement. The patient seeks out the services of a physician, and the physician accepts the patient for treatment. During this relationship, health information is gathered and exchanged between the two parties. Trust between the physician and patient is essential for the sharing of sensitive health information. Without trust in the relationship, confidentiality would be undermined. The principle of confidentiality requires physicians to keep all patients' health information private. When a patient understands their information will be kept private, he/she will be encouraged to seek out care and be open during the visit about his/her health condition. This is especially important with information pertaining to diseases of psychiatric, sexual, or drug/alcohol origins.

## Educating Healthcare Staff on Privacy and Confidentiality Issues
### Required Compliance with HIPAA Regulations

Any covered entity is required to comply with the Health Insurance Portability and Accountability Act (HIPAA). How is a covered entity defined? A covered entity is defined as a healthcare provider, health plans, healthcare clearinghouses, and business associates (e.g., entities who transmit protected health information [PHI] data or vendors who offer the services of personal health records). Compliance with HIPAA regulations means the covered entity has taken measures to protect the privacy and security of their patients' health information.

### Importance of Healthcare Staff Being Knowledgeable of Privacy and Confidentiality Issues

HIPAA, also known as the Privacy Rule, is a federal law. It is important for healthcare staff to understand their role in ensuring compliance with this law. Compliance with HIPAA is not the responsibility of physicians or healthcare administrative staff only. Protecting the privacy and security of health information is the responsibility of all healthcare workers, whether they serve in a clinical role or a non-clinical role. Therefore, all healthcare staff must be knowledgeable of the following (at a minimum):

- what information is protected
- when it is appropriate to disclose protected health information
- the types of healthcare information that is considered sensitive with more strict regulations
- the types of penalties (criminal and civil) for confidentiality breaches
- the consequences of breaches to include disciplinary action, loss of job, and lawsuits

## CONTINUING EDUCATION REGARDING HEALTHCARE PRIVACY

Training for providers regarding privacy is not optional for healthcare entities. HIPAA requires that all staff (including contracted individuals and volunteers) must be trained in maintaining the privacy and confidentiality of protected health information. The training must be provided to new staff members within a reasonable time of their employment date (most employers provide the training as part of on-boarding of new staff members). Documentation that training occurred must be maintained for each staff member. Policies and procedures (P&Ps) pertaining to privacy and confidentiality must be kept current, and when changes are made to the P&Ps, subsequent training must be carried out. Confidentiality/privacy training must also be conducted annually for all employees in order to keep employees up-to-date with current privacy practices.

# Recognizing and Reporting Privacy Issues or Violations

## HEALTHCARE PRIVACY VIOLATIONS

Healthcare privacy violations may come in many different forms. Some examples of violations would be:

- Posting protected health information (PHI) on a social media site.
- Inappropriate access of a patient's electronic medical record when not involved in his/her care.
- Inappropriate access of a high-profile account (e.g., politician, movie star) and release of that information for financial profit.
- Failure to dispose of printed PHI in a shredder and instead disposed of in a regular trashcan.
- Leaving a telephone message pertaining to PHI without permission to do so.
- Faxing PHI to the wrong number.
- Conversation between healthcare staff about a patient's case in a public place within earshot of the public (e.g., hospital cafeteria)

## REPORTING PRIVACY VIOLATIONS INTERNALLY

When an employee suspects a privacy violation, he/she should immediately alert his/her manager. If this is not an appropriate option (e.g., the manager may be the violator), the Privacy Officer and/or Corporate Compliance Officer (CCO) should be notified through email or by calling the healthcare entity's employee Compliance Hotline. An option to report a suspected privacy violation anonymously must be made available to employees, such as a Compliance Hotline. CCOs or Privacy Officers will investigate further the suspected violations through interviews, interrogations, and computer analysis. The determination to proceed with seeking the advice of legal counsel will be made, and reporting of violations may be necessary depending upon the severity of the violation. Disciplinary action, up to and including termination of the violator's employment, may be an appropriate course of action.

## REPORTING HEALTHCARE PRIVACY VIOLATIONS TO REGULATORY BODIES

Anyone can file a privacy or security violation complaint with the Office for Civil Rights (OCR). The complainant, as mentioned, can be anyone, such as a healthcare employee who works for the entity where the violation has allegedly occurred, or someone not affiliated with the healthcare entity. The complaint can be filed in writing, via fax, through email, or via the OCR portal. When filing the complaint, the following information should be provided: name of the complainant, contact information, and details of the suspected violation. After receiving the complaint, the OCR will investigate further and will only take action if they determine that rights were violated and the complaint was filed within 180 days of its occurrence. The OCR will issue a letter describing their investigation and they may issue corrective action for the healthcare entity or impose civil monetary penalties.

## Penalties Associated with Healthcare Privacy Violations

The American Recovery and Reinvestment Act of 2009 established the civil penalties associated with healthcare privacy violations of HIPAA. The penalties can be as follows:

| Violation | Minimum Penalty | Maximum Penalty |
|---|---|---|
| Unintentional disclosure of PHI | $100 per violation up to $25,000 annually for repeat violations | $50,000 per violation up to $1.5 million annually |
| Reasonable cause, not due to intentional neglect | $1,000 per violation up to $100,000 for repeat violations | $50,000 per violation up to $1.5 million annually |
| Due to intentional neglect but violation corrected | $10,000 per violation up to $250,000 for repeat violations | $50,000 per violation up to $1.5 million annually |
| Due to intentional neglect and violation not corrected | $50,000 per violation up to $1.5 million annually | $50,000 per violation up to $1.5 million annually |

# Maintaining a Secure Work Environment

## Securing Health Information

Part of HIPAA addresses the Security Rule. In order for providers to comply with HIPAA's Security Rule, a risk analysis must be conducted in order to identify and implement measures to ensure the security of electronic protected health information (e-PHI). The primary purpose of the risk analysis tool is to thoroughly assess potential risks and vulnerabilities to the privacy, integrity, and accessibility of a provider's e-PHI. For identified risks and vulnerabilities, a provider must initiate a risk management process. The best practice a provider can follow is to implement an integrated risk analysis and management process that is a continuous process that assesses new technologies and operations as they are initiated.

## Safeguards for PHI

PHI must be protected by administrative, physical, and technical safeguards. Administrative safeguards refer to policies and procedures that address PHI security as well as a security risk assessment and risk management plans. Physical safeguards can be in the form of facility access controls to information technology (IT) areas (e.g., badge-only access), restrictions of computer station access, use, and security, and hardware and media controls (e.g., how to properly dispose of IT media, how to backup IT media). Technical safeguards are safeguards that are integrated into IT systems to protect access to IT data. For example, individual authentication ensures the person needing access is a valid requestor.

## Phishing Emails

Phishing emails are targeted emails aimed at stealing information. Healthcare entities receive phishing emails just like any other business entity. Phishing emails can appear in any of the following formats:

- Emails with suspicious hyperlinks and/or attachments
- Poor spelling and/or grammar
- Unrealistic threat such as being turned over to authorities if not compliant with request
- Request for money
- Request for personal information

Healthcare entities must be proactive in preventing the phishing emails and their associated effects of privacy breaches. New employee education and annual reminders to staff about ways to prevent becoming a victim of phishing emails is important. Staff should also be assessed by the healthcare's IT department through the means of sending a fake phishing email and assessing how many employees fall for the trick.

## Passcodes in PHI Security

Passcodes or passwords are the simplest form of security for PHI. However, they can also be the easiest to crack by those with the wrong intentions. Maintaining passcodes can be frustrating for the user due to the many different passcode requirements for different systems. Healthcare entities should have effective policies and procedures (P&Ps) in place that address the requirements for passcodes. The P&Ps should incorporate at a minimum the following points to prevent passcode cracking:

- Avoid use of words written backwards.
- Avoid use of personal information.
- Use passcodes with long lengths, complex width (meaning use of symbols, and not just alpha characters), and complex depth (e.g., passcodes that are not easily guessed).
- Use encryption.
- Instead of writing down passcodes, write down phrases that will jog the memory of the passcode.
- Change passcodes on a frequent basis.
- Lock accounts with more than 3 unsuccessful attempts.

## Developing Strong Passcodes

Passcodes are one essential way to secure PHI. They are not fail-proof, however, to hackers. Following are key tips regarding strong passcodes:

- Create passwords that cannot be easily guessed.
- Change passwords frequently.
- Do not use the same password for multiple systems.
- Use a combination of capitalization, symbols, numbers, and alpha characters.
- Do not always capitalize the first letter of the passcode; rather, capitalize an alpha character in the middle or at the end of the passcode.
- Never use part of the username as part of the password.
- Use a word in its numerical equivalent of a telephone pad (e.g., flash would convert to 35274).
- Use two words separated by symbols.
- Use the first letter of each word in a phrase (e.g., I love McDonald's tea becomes ILMT).

# Minimum Necessary Documentation and Release of Information

## Minimum Necessary

In the healthcare world of PHI, "minimum necessary" is a common phrase. Minimum necessary can be defined as: The amount of patient information that is released or accessed only when there is a legitimate need to know. When a legitimate request is validated, only the minimum necessary amount of information needed to perform a job function should be provided or accessed. It is important for healthcare employees to understand that accessing their own health information (without going through the proper channels of a properly authorized release) is prohibited. This same prohibition applies to accessing the health information of friends, relatives, or coworkers, unless there is a legitimate need to know. Software programs are rather sophisticated and capable of identifying inappropriate accesses based upon an employee's name and address. For example, if an employee accesses a neighbor's health information, the software will identify the access as a probable inappropriate access based solely upon the employee's address/locale.

## Measures Enforcing Access to Only Minimal Necessary Information

Access to minimum necessary information means healthcare employees may only have access to PHI for which there is a legitimate need to know. Healthcare privacy departments are tasked with ensuring PHI is kept secure, and for those instances when the privacy has been breached, it the privacy department's responsibility to investigate further and coordinate disciplinary action with healthcare managers. Some examples of measures a privacy department could implement for the control of access to PHI might be:

- tracking of electronic requests
- analysis of electronic PHI accesses
- investigation of verbal or emailed complaints about potential improper accesses
- application of software packages aimed at identifying improper accesses

## Required Elements of a Written Authorization to Release Information

When a patient requests release of his or her health information to himself or herself or a third party, a written authorization is required. A written authorization to release information should include the following components:

- Name of the healthcare entity releasing the information
- Name of the individual to receive the information
- Patient's full name and other identifying data (e.g., address, date of birth)
- Purpose for needing the information
- Type of information to be released with specified dates of service (e.g., discharge summary, operative report)
- Authorization expiration date
- Authorization revocation statement
- Patient's or legal representative's signature and date

## Prohibition of Redisclosure

When a healthcare entity releases patient information to a third party, a statement should be included in the release that prohibits redisclosure. Once the health information is released, the releasing healthcare entity has no control over what happens to the information from that point forward. Therefore, it is necessary for the releasing healthcare entity to include a statement that prohibits redisclosure. This statement informs the recipient of their obligation in maintaining privacy of the patient's health information. The statement should also instruct the recipient to only use the information for the intended purpose noted in the release.

## Effect of Court Orders/Subpoenas on Releasing of Health Information

When a court order/subpoena is received in a health information management (HIM) department, it must be obeyed. The court order/subpoena will instruct the HIM director of which healthcare documents must be submitted. Upon receipt of the subpoena, it should be assessed for its validity (e.g., name and location of the court, signature of the court clerk, court seal). All court orders/subpoenas should be logged in, and HIM personnel should determine whether the requested records even exist. Requested records should be assessed for completeness, followed by

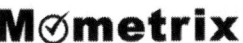

copying of the completed documents onto an electronic medium (e.g., CD). A statement should be included with the copies to testify that the information is a certified copy.

## Protecting Electronic Documentation

### ENCRYPTION

Encryption is a security method or control that provides protection for confidential information. Encryption applies a mathematical algorithm that scrambles the data into a format that cannot be deciphered by people or computerized systems. The scrambled text is also known as ciphertext. Encryption is a reversible process, meaning that the scrambled test can be unscrambled back into its original form. When the data are unscrambled, the method is referred to as decryption. In brief, encryption and decryption go hand-in-hand, and both functions require a cryptographic key that applies one or the other function. The cryptographic key must be kept secret in order for encryption to be fail-proof and confidentiality of the information protected.

### MEDICAL IDENTITY THEFT

Medical identity theft is on the rise. The impact upon patients can be devastating because the breach may result in criminals maximizing health benefits of the victim's insurance plan, or the criminal may be successful in obtaining prescription drugs. In some cases, thieves hold health information ransom, demanding large sums of money to return the health information to the patient or healthcare entity. HIM professionals should be involved in mitigating the risks associated with medical identity theft. HIM professionals can build awareness that medical identity is a patient safety issue. They can provide staff education regarding how to identify fraudulent activity. They can also work with IT in mitigating phishing scams and initiating valid passcode applications. HIM professionals can also assist in identifying fraudulent activity through data analysis and the performance of proactive audits.

### CYBERSECURITY

While IT departments are the key individuals responsible for the security of health information, HIM professionals should be involved since they are knowledgeable of information workflows. Healthcare entities are wise to use their IT staff as well as HIM staff to proactively implement cybersecurity plans for the purpose of preventing cybercriminal activities. A cybersecurity plan should include a risk assessment of all software applications used by the healthcare entity. The risk assessment should look for protection gaps, and the identified vulnerable systems should be patched to close the weakness. Encryption is another vital method that should be used in the fight against cyber theft. All workstations and portable mediums should be encrypted. Encryption is effective in that it scrambles the data so that they cannot be deciphered by people or electronic systems.

Cybersecurity is a method aimed at protecting information collected and maintained in the culture of information technology from cybercriminal activity. Cybersecurity is a plan that focuses on preventing information theft or information attacks (e.g., viruses, malware). Cybercriminals may steal health information for the purpose of maximizing health benefits from the victim's insurance plan, or for the purpose of obtaining prescription drugs, or for the purpose of holding health information ransom, demanding large sums of money to return the health information to the patient or healthcare entity. The intention behind information attacks from viruses or malware may be from disgruntled employees or terrorists, sometimes referred to as hacktivists. Because of the numerous cyber threats increasing daily in the healthcare world, cybersecurity is an absolute necessity to protect patients' health information.

## TOP CYBERSECURITY CONCERNS

Healthcare cybersecurity threats take many different forms. Some of the most obvious are: phishing emails, viruses, malware, and ransomware. All of these threats are intended to "wage war" against the attacked entity. A disgruntled healthcare employee, angry patient, or frustrated stakeholder/business associate may be the party who bring about such attacks. Other cyber threats may come in the form of biomedical devices aimed at harming patients' lives or through unsecured cloud storage. In some cases, health information may be inadvertently stored in a cloud, and the cloud may not be secure, or information may be stored in a "smart" device that has not been secured by the healthcare organization. Lack of antivirus software or intrusion prevention software can also put portable devices at risk. Each of these cybersecurity concerns need to be assessed by all healthcare entities in order to implement effective security measures.

## HEALTH INFORMATION EXCHANGE (HIE)

Health Information Exchange (HIE) is the movement of PHI between organizations, such as hospitals and physician's offices. Through HIE processes, medical information is shared electronically, and the result is a fast communication of information that improves the quality, safety, and cost of patient care. The Office of the National Coordinator for Health Information Technology's (ONC) Office of Science & Technology (OST) is responsible for the development of nationally recognized HIE standards. The purpose of the standards is to promote consistency between all healthcare providers in how information is exchanged. Providers are encouraged to participate in HIE processes in order to provide more effective, efficient health care.

## SECURELY TRANSFERRING EMAILS AND ELECTRONIC FILES

It is possible to transfer emails and electronic files containing PHI securely. There are steps involved in order to ensure the security of transmitted information. One step is to encrypt email communications. The easiest encryption method for email communications in Microsoft Outlook is to access the Trust Center under the Tools menu and select "encrypt contents and attachments of outgoing messages." The recipient will need the sender's digital ID in order to decode the message. This same process can be accomplished through services that provide encryption keys and/or digital certificates. Files can also be secured through accessing Internet sites that have an HTTPS address, and not just an HTTP address. The "S" implies that the site is secure, which is advantageous for the use and transfer of sensitive files, such as PHI.

# Record Retention and Destruction

## MEDICAL RECORD OWNERSHIP

The medical record is a compilation of all written, printed, or electronic information recorded by a healthcare provider as he/she communicates with the patient during the treatment or period. Since two parties are involved in the process of creating the record of collected information, the question is raised: Who owns the medical record? The understanding in the HIM profession is that the medical record is the property of the provider who maintains it. The information maintained in the medical record can be accessed or obtained by the patient or his/her legal representative at any time by going through the appropriate channels of releasing the information.

## HEALTHCARE RETENTION POLICIES

Healthcare retention policies must be a requirement for healthcare providers. A formal plan of retention or a record retention schedule should be developed and maintained by the HIM director. This plan should define active and inactive records/information. Statute of limitations should be addressed in the policies as well as the requirements set forth by regulatory bodies such as the federal Conditions of Participation (CoPs), the Federal Register, the Joint Commission, state regulations, and the American Health Information Management Association (AHIMA) regulations. Record retention policies should also outline the method of destruction or archival of health information in its various mediums.

## REGULATORY BODIES PROVIDING GUIDANCE APPLICABLE TO THE RETENTION OF HEALTHCARE INFORMATION

Retention of healthcare information or medical records is regulated by various external agencies. The federal Conditions of Participation (CoPs) is one of the most prominent regulations governing this aspect of health information. The Federal Register is another source that provides guidance pertaining to retention requirements. State-specific requirements exist as well. The Joint Commission, a healthcare accrediting body, also weighs in on retention requirements, and the American Health Information Management Association (AHIMA) does also. Between the federal, state, Joint Commission, and AHIMA's guidance, each healthcare entity must follow the guidance that is more restrictive. Retention also hinges upon whether records are deemed active or inactive, with active meaning the information is still being consulted on a regular basis, and inactive meaning the information is rarely accessed.

## LEGAL HEALTH RECORD

The legal health record is a compilation of individually identifiable data as well as the documentation of services rendered to a patient by the healthcare provider. Each healthcare entity must define in their policies and bylaws the content of the legal record. The content of the legal record may be composed of both paper and electronic documents. The content of the legal record must also comply with standards set forth by external agencies, such as the Joint Commission, CMS, HIPAA, and federal and state regulations. The legal health record serves the purposes of patient care, administrative, business, and financial purposes. Additionally, it is considered a legal document that is submissible as evidence in court proceedings.

## DESTROYING HEALTH INFORMATION

Health information may be destroyed when in compliance with federal and state regulations. Destruction would be applicable to inactive records only, and the following information should never be destroyed: basic information such as admission and discharge dates, responsible physician names, diagnoses and operations, discharge summaries, operative reports, and pathology reports. Health information of minors should not be destroyed until after the period of their minority has passed plus any time pertaining to statute of limitations has passed. Disease, operative, and physician indices should be kept for a period of 5 to 10 years, depending upon state regulations. Birth and death certificates should be maintained permanently.

## LIFE CYCLE OF A HEALTH RECORD

The life cycle of a health record is composed of four parts: creation, utilization, maintenance, and destruction. A record cannot exist without the creation of information; hence, the first phase in the life cycle. Creation of the health information happens for the purpose of using the information. The information collected helps to guide the healthcare practitioners in the best treatment possible for the patient through this communication tool. When an active date of service is over, the record must still be maintained according to federal and state retention standards. The maintenance time frame varies depending on state regulations, but at some point in time after no further treatment activity, the record is destroyed. Destruction policies and procedures must indicate the appropriate methods of destruction for each type of medium that contains the health information (e.g., paper, microfilm). Electronic data would most likely be archived instead of destroyed.

# Information Blocking

The information blocking rule allows patients to have control over who can access or use their electronic health information (EHI), with eight exceptions. The first five exceptions allow a healthcare provider to block information to a patient, whereas the last three still require access to be provided, but under certain alternative procedures. These eight exceptions are as follows:

- Preventing harm
- Protecting privacy
- Protecting the security of EHI
- Infeasibility (i.e., not having the technological capabilities or legal rights to fulfill a request)
- Information technology performance (i.e., systems are temporarily unavailable)
- Content and manner (i.e., being technically unable to fulfill the request in the manner requested)
- Unpaid fees
- Licensing

The information blocking rule also outlines penalties, which include disincentives to healthcare providers, and a complaint process when the rule is not followed.

## RISKS AND BENEFITS OF INFORMATION BLOCKING

The information blocking rule was designed to ultimately benefit patients. Patients can not only use and access their EHI almost immediately, but they can also do so on apps so their information is located in one hub instead of existing within multiple portals. Additionally, patients no longer need to provide written consent in order for one healthcare entity to exchange EHI with another healthcare entity, which makes it easier for healthcare professionals to get a better idea of a patient's health status and to provide the best treatment options. On the other hand, because the information blocking rule makes healthcare more transparent, healthcare professionals should ensure that what they are documenting is accurate and not offensive. They, along with their staff, will also need to learn how to comply with these new regulations and what penalties are imposed for information blocking.

# CCA Practice Test #1

Want to take this practice test in an online interactive format? Check out the bonus page, which includes interactive practice questions and much more: **mometrix.com/bonus948/certcodeasso**

1. What is (are) the appropriate International Classification of Diseases, 10th Revision (ICD-10) code(s) for symptoms of nausea with vomiting?
   a. R11.0
   b. R11.10
   c. R11.2
   d. R11.0, R11.10

2. What is the appropriate ICD-10 code for the diagnosis of a malignant neoplasm of the right male breast located in the upper-inner quadrant?
   a. C50.211
   b. C50.221
   c. C50.411
   d. C50.421

3. A 55-year-old female undergoes surgery to upgrade her single-chamber pacemaker system to a dual-chamber pacemaker system. Select the CPT code(s) for this procedure.
   a. 33249, 33225
   b. 33228
   c. 33241, 33249
   d. 33214

4. What does the acronym PHI stand for?
   a. Protected health information
   b. Private health information
   c. Personal health information
   d. Patient health information

5. Which of the following statements regarding healthcare provisions of Medicare is FALSE?
   a. Medicare covers seniors aged 65+.
   b. Medicare is federally and state funded.
   c. Medicare covers select disability services.
   d. Medicare covers end-stage renal disease services.

6. A patient consents to potentially assume financial responsibility for a service or procedure that may be denied by Medicare. What form must the patient fill out?
   a. CMS-1450
   b. ABN
   c. HIPAA
   d. MIPS

7. A 31-year-old female undergoes surgery for a bilateral salpingectomy. Based on your knowledge of medical terminology, select the appropriate descriptors for this procedure.
   a. Repair of fallopian tubes
   b. Removal of fallopian tubes
   c. Repair of uterus
   d. Removal of uterus

8. What general information about a patient's health history CANNOT be gleaned from the SOAP notes of his or her past visits to the physician's office?
   a. Subjective and objective descriptions of the patient's complaint
   b. The physician's assessment of the patient's complaint
   c. The physician's plan for treating the patient's complaint
   d. Prescription information for treating the patient's complaint

9. An obstetrician documents a 34-year-old female in the delivery room with status G2P2 before successfully delivering a healthy baby boy. What does G2P2 indicate?
   a. Two years since last pregnancy, second of two total pregnancies
   b. Two previous pregnancies, two previous vaginal deliveries
   c. Two previous pregnancies, two previous cesarean deliveries
   d. Two previous pregnancies, two previous live births

10. Jason's left leg is quarter-inch shorter than his right leg. His podiatrist orders a custom orthotic shoe insert to make walking more comfortable. In which manual would the code for an orthotic insert be found?
    a. ICD-10-CM
    b. CPT
    c. HCPCS-II
    d. OIG

11. In which category of the ICD-10 would you find an appropriate code for an adult patient's routine visit to see his or her family physician?
    a. Category Z
    b. Category A
    c. Category K
    d. Category R

12. A radiologist is performing a procedure requiring the careful maneuver of imaging equipment and contrast material among several different arterial vessels. Which appendix in the CPT codebook best guides proper code selection for this procedure?
    a. Category III – vascular imaging is a new and emerging technology.
    b. Appendix A – different blood vessels will require the use of different modifiers.
    c. Appendix C – the coder must study clinical examples of this highly complex procedure before assigning codes.
    d. Appendix L – knowledge of vascular families is crucial to coding accurately in this field.

13. Mr. Greenbriar was admitted as an inpatient for emergency treatment of an end-stage renal disease flare-up. The day after his admission, his personal physician comes to the hospital for a checkup and chart review. Select the appropriate E/M code series for his physician's visit.
    a. Office or other outpatient services (99201–99215)
    b. Subsequent hospital care (99231–99233)
    c. Initial hospital care (99221–99223)
    d. Initial observation care (99218–99220)

14. A 43-year-old male is rushed to the emergency department after sustaining life-threatening injuries from a car wreck. Upon arrival, he is immediately approved for critical care services. The physician administering care spends a total of 105 minutes stabilizing and treating the patient that day. Select the appropriate E/M code(s) for this service.
    a. 99291, 99292×2
    b. 99291, 99292
    c. 99283
    d. 99285

15. Which of the following statements is TRUE regarding the correct coding of hospital discharge services?
    a. When someone is discharged from inpatient services on the same date as admission, the coder consults E/M series 99234–99236.
    b. Code 99239 is used only for discharge services that also include a final examination as part of the discharge procedure.
    c. Codes 99238 and 99239 can be used for patients being discharged from nursing facility care.
    d. A discharge service of 30 minutes is coded 99239.

16. Based on your knowledge of the three pillars of E/M services (i.e., history, exam, and medical decision making), which of these patient evaluation components does NOT belong with the others?
    a. Chief complaint
    b. History of present illness
    c. Review of systems
    d. Level of risk

17. Kendra, a collegiate soccer player, presents for her second appointment at Dr. Yakamoto's office to discuss treatment options for her torn meniscus. Her first appointment, just last week, was a consultation visit at the request of her personal physician, and Dr. Yakamoto agreed to take responsibility for her care at the end of that first visit. What E/M code is appropriate for Kendra's second visit?
    a. 99243
    b. 99254
    c. 99203
    d. 99213

18. Which of the following E/M service codes is appropriate for a healthy 8-year-old boy's routine checkup with his pediatrician?
    a. 99201
    b. 99393
    c. 99211
    d. 99383

19. An anesthesiologist with knowledge of coding in his field is double-checking a new coder's modifiers for an anesthesia service he performed yesterday. He also teaches and trains anesthesiology residents, one of whom worked with him under his direct guidance and supervision during this same procedure. The coder's documentation for anesthesiology services includes the head modifier QY, with a total modifier combination of QY-QS-P1 for the surgical procedure. How would the physician approach the coder about the accuracy of the coding work?
    a. The physician would have no comments because the head modifier for total services rendered (QY) is correct.
    b. The physician would tell the coder to move the modifier QY to the end of the sequence (i.e., QS-P1-QY).
    c. The physician would tell the coder to replace modifier QY with modifier GC for a sequence of GC-QS-P1.
    d. The physician would tell the coder to replace modifier QY with modifier GC and to reorder the sequence with P1-GC-QS.

20. A 66-year-old female shatters her right tibia due to a spiral fracture while skiing. After an initial evaluation in the emergency department, she is immediately admitted to surgery with Dr. Rigo for an intramedullary implant. In her first 24 hours of recovery, she develops a rare reaction to the implant in which the pressure inside her leg has become dangerously high. She is promptly readmitted to the operating room for Dr. Rigo to surgically remedy the pressure caused by the implant. Using your knowledge of Medicare's global surgical package provisions, what modifier is needed for coding this second surgery?
    a. 76
    b. 77
    c. 78
    d. 79

21. A 34-year-old woman presents to her obstetrician-gynecologist (OB-GYN) to drain a large cyst on her vulva that had developed as a result of shaving. During the lidocaine injection, the patient screams in pain, but tells the doctor to continue the procedure. After waiting a few minutes for numbing to occur, the physician attempts to break the surface of the cyst with a scalpel several times, but the patient's distress due to pain only worsens. After the patient turns down a second dose of lidocaine through tears, the doctor immediately discontinues the procedure. The patient is then calmed and discharged with an antibiotic. How should the incision and drainage procedure be reported?
    a. The incision and drainage procedure is not reported.
    b. The incision and drainage procedure is reported with modifier 52.
    c. The incision and drainage procedure is reported with modifier 53.
    d. The incision and drainage procedure is reported, but without modifiers.

22. A healthy patient whose brother needs a kidney transplant presents to the hospital for surgery as a matching donor. The admitting physician performs a comprehensive history, a comprehensive exam, and medical decision making that is highly complex. What is the appropriate code for this encounter?

    a. 99222
    b. 99223
    c. 99233
    d. 99236

23. Dr. Minnick, an OB-GYN, is called to an emergency delivery of a premature baby with known cardiopulmonary abnormalities. Dr. Minnick immediately requests that his colleague Dr. Arapoglou be on standby while he delivers the baby, due to the likely case that he will need cardiopulmonary care upon delivery. Once both physicians are present, Dr. Minnick delivers the baby within 10 minutes. As expected, the baby cannot breathe properly upon arrival and quickly slips into unconsciousness. Thankfully, Dr. Arapoglou manages to resuscitate him. The newborn is then immediately transferred out of the birthing room to the neonatal intensive care unit via the pediatric transport team. What code(s) should be reported for Dr. Arapoglou's encounter with the newborn?

    a. 99360
    b. 99465
    c. 99465, 99464
    d. 99465, 99360

24. After attempting suicide, Denise is admitted to the local psychiatric treatment center. She will remain there under 24/7 supervision until she is no longer deemed a threat to herself or others. What code is used for her admission?

    a. 99220
    b. 99223
    c. 99306
    d. 99310

25. An 18-year-old patient presents to a minute clinic for a sore throat. The physician who sees her gathers an expanded problem-focused history and performs an expanded problem-focused exam. The medical decision making is straightforward. What is the appropriate code for this encounter?

    a. 99202
    b. 99213
    c. 99201
    d. 99215

26. Patient Report: "General: Sofia is alert & very pleasant for a 5-year-old. NAD. Eyes: PERRLA. Neck, throat: no inflammation or anomalies detected upon palpation. Chest: RRR. Abdomen: tender, healthy upon auscultation. Joints: responsive reflexes; good ROM. Overall: developing well since the first visit last year; next annual to be scheduled today." What code should be assigned for this encounter?

    a. 99393
    b. 99383
    c. 99201
    d. 99211

27. Dan is a 25-year-old working in the auto racing industry. His father just died of liver failure and was a known alcoholic. Shortly after his dad's passing, Dan gets a DNA test and discovers that he is genetically predisposed to hepatic steatosis. He decides to start seeing a specialist regularly in order to develop strategies that result in drastically cutting back on his alcohol consumption. He describes himself as a "heavy drinker" at his first appointment, but his medical record shows no documentation of any known diseases or health issues. Which code appropriately documents Dan's initial 30-minute visit?

   a. 99385
   b. 99408
   c. 99409
   d. 99402

28. A patient who until now was in remission from lung cancer appears to have developed a new growth in her right lung. Dr. McKinnon performs a thoracotomy with a diagnostic biopsy of the nodule in question. Shortly after the procedure, Dr. McKinnon performs a repeat thoracotomy to control an unexpected postoperative hemorrhage due to a small tear near the initial place of surgery. What is the code and/or code-modifier combination necessary to correctly document this second procedure?

   a. 32097
   b. 32098
   c. 32120-78
   d. 32120-76

29. A landscape worker was throwing a large tree branch into the wood chipper on his truck. He unexpectedly lost his balance, causing his safety glasses to slip off. Consequently, his eyes were scratched with a flurry of fine woodchip dust before he fell onto some decorative rocks and sliced the skin on both of his right eyelids. Dr. Tardy is now repairing the lacerations in the operating room. Due to the extensive prevalence of woodchip dust, however, the site of injury required an unusual amount of flushing and cleaning for 20 extra minutes before he could start the repair of the skin itself. Overall, 2.8 cm of skin was sutured in an intermediate-level repair. What codes accurately document the nature of the surgery performed by Dr. Tardy?

   a. 12051, 12052-22
   b. 12052-22-E3-E4
   c. 67930-22-E3-E4
   d. 67930-E3-E4, 67938

30. A patient with known skin sensitivity presents for a follow-up appointment with his family physician to assess the healing of the warts that were removed from his forehead the previous week in the office. After a quick check-in, the physician determines that no further action is needed. The patient, however, complains of painful urination that started three days prior that hasn't subsided. After checking his chart, the physician orders a urinalysis to determine if the patient has a urinary tract infection (UTI). What code(s) and/or code-modifier combinations correctly document the E/M side of this encounter?

   a. 99212
   b. 99212, 99212-25
   c. 99212×2
   d. 99212, 99212-59

31. Christine is scheduled for spine surgery in a month, but she continues to experience terrible lumbago symptoms on a daily basis. She presents to the spine clinic for a steroid injection to help make her pain manageable before the procedure to repair a displaced lumbar disc, an injury she sustained in a recent car wreck. Select the correct set of diagnosis code sequences for her visit.
    a. M54.40, G89.11
    b. M51.26, G89.11
    c. G89.11, M51.26
    d. G89.11, M54.5

32. Carlos presents to an outpatient facility with instructions to undergo some routine lab tests as part of his annual physical he had earlier that day: a basic metabolic panel and a general health panel. Select the appropriate ICD-10 and CPT codes for the lab encounter.
    a. Z00.00, 80047, 80050
    b. Z00.01, 80053, 80050
    c. Z00.00, 80053, 80050
    d. Z00.01, 80048, 80050

33. Mary takes her mother, Gertrude, to an audiology center. Gertrude has been struggling with hearing for about one month and she occasionally experiences vertigo. Gertrude's physician suspects Ménière's disease, so he referred her for a comprehensive audiometry evaluation of her left ear. Select the appropriate ICD-10 and CPT codes for Gertrude's encounter.
    a. H91.22, R42, 92557
    b. H81.02, 92557-52
    c. H81.02, 92557
    d. H91.22, R42, 92557-52

34. A patient with human immunodeficiency virus (HIV) is admitted to the hospital with a diagnosis of bilateral otitis media and HIV-related Kaposi's sarcoma of the left lung. What is the correct sequence of diagnostic codes for this patient?
    a. H66.90, B20, C46.51
    b. B20, C46.52, H66.93
    c. B20, C46.52, H66.90
    d. B20, Z21, C46.51, H66.93

35. A healthy 33-year-old male undergoes a laparoscopic cholecystectomy procedure under general anesthesia. The anesthesia was personally provided by an anesthesiologist while the surgeon performed the procedure. What is the correct sequence of procedural codes for the anesthesiologist and the surgeon?
    a. 00790-AA-P1; 47563
    b. 00790-AD-P1; 47564
    c. 00790-AD-P1; 47562
    d. 00790-AA-P1; 47562

36. Mr. Jeong, a 67-year-old male with Medicare, is at the outpatient surgery center for a colonoscopy screening. Despite his age, he is considered a patient of low-risk status for developing colorectal cancer. What is the appropriate code for this encounter?

   a. 45378
   b. 45378-33
   c. G0105
   d. G0121

37. George, a patient with Medicare, is at the outpatient surgery center. As a past colorectal cancer survivor, he continues to be at high risk for recurrence. During his colonoscopy screening for colorectal cancer, the doctor notices an abnormality and performs a biopsy. What is/are the appropriate code(s) for his encounter?

   a. G0105, 45380
   b. G0121
   c. 45380
   d. 45380, 45378

38. What is the appropriate DRG code for a discharged patient with alpha thalassemia as a major secondary complication or comorbidity?

   a. 808
   b. 811
   c. 812
   d. 813

39. What is the DRG code for a discharged patient whose prostate was excised via his urethra in the operating room without a primary or secondary complication or comorbidity?

   a. 707
   b. 708
   c. 713
   d. 714

40. A coder documents CPT codes for a two-part procedure in the spine clinic. Both procedures, although similar, have different ambulatory payment classification (APC) numbers, 5462 and 5464, respectively. Both APCs are status J1 codes. Based on Medicare's reimbursement policies, how should the coder submit the claim?

   a. The coder should submit both CPT codes, but only one APC code.
   b. The coder should submit both CPT codes with their respective APC codes.
   c. The coder should submit both CPT codes without their APC codes.
   d. The coder should only submit the APC codes.

41. APC status level indicator C is only ever seen in outpatient center claims. What does this indicator stand for?

   a. Ambulance services
   b. Partial hospitalization
   c. Clinic or emergency department visit
   d. Inpatient procedures

42. When consulting the NCCI edit tables, service and procedure codes are grouped together in pairs. Why is this so?
    a. The use of pairs indicates that the codes are interchangeable depending on the circumstances.
    b. The use of pairs indicates codes that may or may not be reported together.
    c. The use of pairs represents codes for the same procedure that differentiate between simple and complex.
    d. The use of pairs shows which new code is being reviewed to replace an old code.

43. Denise is unsure if procedure codes 12345 and 54321 can be reported together or not. She consults the latest NCCI edits and notices that both codes are grouped together with a correct coding modifier indicator of 1. What does this mean for Denise's coding decision?
    a. Denise cannot report the codes together in her claim.
    b. Denise can report the codes together in her claim.
    c. Denise can report the codes together in her claim, but only with a modifier.
    d. Denise can choose one code or the other for her claim.

44. A new coder specializing in orthopedics reviews the NCCI edits and learns that they designate CPT surgical code pair 27889 and 69990 as 0. Which rationale would make the most sense for this decision?
    a. The use of code 69990 is not necessary for the procedure.
    b. Code 69990 is modifier-51 exempt.
    c. Codes 27889 and 69990 are both add-on codes.
    d. Codes 27889 and 69990 are mutually exclusive in all orthopedic surgeries.

45. A young dermatologist performing surgery soon asks his coder about the reimbursement rules surrounding a numbing technique that he is considering, which currently corresponds to code 0230T. After doing some research, the coder notices that it has a 0 designation when paired with the surgery corresponding to CPT code 11042. What would the coder tell the doctor?
    a. The doctor will be reimbursed for the work involving both codes when reported together.
    b. CMS will cover the cost for 0230T, but not the cost for procedure 11042.
    c. Code 0230T is automatically bundled into the reimbursement services for procedure 11042.
    d. CMS will deny the claim if both codes are reported together.

46. For CMS, Title XVIII, §1862(a)(1) of the Social Security Act is crucial for determining the medical necessity of services and/or procedures. These regulations are outlined in the *National Coverage Determinations Manual* and clearly indicate the circumstances under which a service may be reimbursed. Which of the following scenarios demonstrates a medically necessary service?
    a. A healthy patient without a history of cardiac disease calls her primary care provider with concerns about a recent episode of tachycardia. The physician invites her to come in for an electrocardiogram.
    b. A stay-at-home mother accidentally slices her left thumb while in the kitchen. The laceration is a quarter inch deep, and it immediately starts bleeding. She calls 911, and the operator sends an ambulance.
    c. A high school student notices that she cannot see what is written on the chalkboard in her algebra class. She gets her eyes tested and finds out that she has developed astigmatism in both eyes. She is promptly scheduled for laser vision correction surgery.
    d. A 14-year-old male is taken to the dermatologist by his father with complaints of a severe acne breakout on his back. The dermatologist performs an in-office punch biopsy to determine the cause.

47. Mr. Johnson, age 69, is diagnosed with decompression sickness at a Houston emergency department after his first scuba diving class in the Gulf of Mexico. He asked the emergency physician if hyperbaric oxygen (HBO) therapy treatment was available to him, a service a friend of his had received in the same hospital when he also developed the same sickness two years prior. The physician consults the local coverage determination (LCD) index for Texas and learns that this therapy (L35021) was "retired" on 8/27/2020. What does this mean?
    a. Medicare in Texas will cover Mr. Johnson's HBO treatment.
    b. Medicare in Texas will only partially cover Mr. Johnson's HBO treatment.
    c. Medicare in Texas will cover HBO treatment under plan B, but not plan A.
    d. Medicare in Texas no longer covers HBO treatment.

48. Which of the following statements is FALSE regarding submitting claims?
    a. Claims are processed by Medicare administrative contractors.
    b. Claims can include NPIs, but they are not required.
    c. Claims can be submitted electronically through an electronic data interchange.
    d. Claims that have been paid are returned to providers along with their respective remittance advice.

49. Put the following steps in the order in which they typically occur:
   1. ICD-10 and CPT codes are assigned to patient encounter.
   2. The claim is approved.
   3. An e-claim is sent to the patient's insurance company.
   4. The patient is billed for the difference as necessary.
   5. The insurance company pays the provider.
   6. The e-claim is sent to a clearinghouse.
   7. The patient's demographic, insurance, and health code information is entered into the billing system.

   a. 1, 7, 3, 6, 2, 5, 4
   b. 7, 1, 6, 3, 2, 4, 5
   c. 7, 1, 2, 3, 5, 6, 4
   d. 1, 7, 6, 3, 2, 5, 4

50. Eric, an employee in accounts receivable, calls Morgan in patient billing to let her know that Mrs. Fallon has still not paid her medical bill. Depending on the severity of the case (anywhere from mild to delinquent), which of the following is NOT an appropriate course of action for collecting this patient's balance?

   a. Morgan sends Mrs. Fallon an additional statement.
   b. Morgan sends Mrs. Fallon a letter to remind her of the unpaid balance on her account.
   c. Morgan informs Mrs. Fallon that her bill will accrue interest until it is paid in full.
   d. Morgan refers Mrs. Fallon's case to a collections agency.

51. A biller in a small otology practice receives a Medicare Part B claim that has been denied and asks a coding colleague to help her troubleshoot the issue. On the claim, the reason for the denial reads: "Codes submitted are for reporting purposes only." Choose what the coder would likely advise.

   a. "Rewrite your modifier 80 more clearly—it looks like an '8P'."
   b. "Make sure you submit a G code for this audiology service instead of a level II."
   c. "Fill out the CMS-1500 again, but leave box 24 blank."
   d. "You used the wrong form for this patient's cochlear implant consultation—use the UB-04 instead when you resubmit."

52. A patient undergoes a procedure for a laparoscopic oophorectomy. The coder submits the claim with the procedure codes listed as 58661×2. The claim is denied and sent back for correction. Which of the following is the MOST likely reason for the denial?

   a. The procedure was probably unilateral, so two codes aren't necessary.
   b. The procedure was bilateral but wasn't coded appropriately.
   c. The physician had to make two incisions instead of one.
   d. The code can't be doubled for a repair procedure that started out as a diagnostic procedure.

53. A claim is submitted with two service codes: one for a doctor's application of a cast on a patient and one for the same doctor's subsequent care of his patient's fracture. The claim is denied by Medicare. Choose the reason why.

   a. "Insufficient medical necessity."
   b. "Duplicate service."
   c. "The service is not covered by contractor."
   d. "Payment is included in another service previously adjudicated."

54. A claim submitted from a lab facility was denied and returned to the coding/billing department. Select which claim correction would NOT apply to a clinical laboratory claim.
    a. Add the missing Clinical Laboratory Improvement Amendments (CLIA) number.
    b. Remove modifier 91.
    c. Add modifier QW.
    d. Correct the numeric code 81355 to 81535.

55. A patient with Medicare has a procedure done for which Medicare has denied coverage. The patient signed an ABN prior to the procedure. How should the billing department respond?
    a. Call Medicare to justify the denial.
    b. Double-check the submitted claim codes for data errors.
    c. Inform the patient that the procedure was not covered.
    d. Obtain a power of attorney to advocate on behalf of the patient.

56. ABC Insurance is a private health insurance company. Its coding and billing guidelines differ from Medicare's, and claims are often sent back for correction for certain services. Select the code resubmission scenario that MOST likely applies to a private payer such as ABC (versus Medicare).
    a. An HCPCS-II G code is resubmitted as a CPT level I code.
    b. Modifier 50 for procedure XXXX is resubmitted as XXXX-LT, XXXX-RT
    c. A CPT level I code is resubmitted with a CPT level III code.
    d. A CPT level I code is resubmitted as an HCPCS-II T code

57. This sequence was submitted with a claim for an influenza vaccine given to a patient the prior month and was rejected: "90660×2."
Which of the following is the CORRECTED code set for resubmission?
    a. 90471, 90664
    b. 90471-51, 90658
    c. 90473, 90474, 90660
    d. 90473, 90680

58. A doctor's operative report for a cancer patient reads "thyroidectomy with neck dissection." The coder needs more information before submitting her codes to billing. Choose the clarification question that best helps meet her needs.
    a. "Was the procedure unilateral or bilateral?"
    b. "Would you say the neck dissection was limited or radical in nature?"
    c. "Did you also include an isthmectomy?"
    d. "Would you consider the thyroid removal as total or subtotal?"

59. A physician documents that he administered buprenorphine/naloxone to a patient today. Select the most logical question that a coder would ask to clarify the doctor's notes.
    a. "Was the medication delivered orally?"
    b. "Did the patient have a preexisting implant?"
    c. "How many doses were administered?"
    d. "What was the total dosage of buprenorphine in milligrams?"

**60.** An orthopedist has a list of medications that he is considering for a patient with chronic knee pain. He asks a nurse to collect all pertinent information from the patient's record to assist his decision. Which of the following pieces of patient data would be LEAST likely to apply to this scenario?
   a. The patient's psychiatric history
   b. The patient's current medication list and allergies
   c. The patient's alcohol and tobacco use
   d. The patient's chest x-rays

**61.** Which of the following pieces of patient data is considered PHI under HIPAA?
   a. The patient's full name
   b. The patient's age
   c. The patient's date of birth (DOB)
   d. The patient's medical conditions

**62.** According to AHIMA, policy making with regard to clearly defining what specifically constitutes patient legal health records versus designated record sets presents major problem-solving issues for health organizations. Although there is no one-size-fits-all definition for either, some subcategories of data can generally be deemed as being outside the scope of both record types. Keeping this in mind, which of the following pieces of subdata WOULD be included in designated health record sets?
   a. A psychotherapist's notes during patient sessions
   b. Notes from a meeting between the covered entity and its attorney regarding legal disputes with patients
   c. The patient's claims and billing records
   d. Quality indicator/quality measure reports involving the patient's medical data

**63.** AHIMA defines administrative data as *"patient-identifiable data* used for administrative, regulatory, healthcare operation, and payment (financial) purposes." What is the reason such data would not be classified as PHI and therefore part of a patient-designated record under HIPAA?
   a. Unlike PHI, patient-identifiable data cannot be accessed across digital interfaces.
   b. Patient-identifiable data are heavily encrypted by law; PHI is not because it is shareable.
   c. Not all patient-identifiable data pose risks to patient privacy.
   d. Administrative data can only be accessed by top OIG officials who run reports with data submitted anonymously.

**64.** Select the best characterization of what would constitute a quantitative deficiency in a patient's medical record.
   a. There are crucial data fields in the patient record that are missing or incomplete.
   b. There are numerical errors in the patient's record (e.g., a blood pressure reading or a weight/body mass index recording during a routine checkup).
   c. The crucial data fields in the patient records are complete but contain some careless errors.
   d. The quantity (amount) of patient data is low when compared to other patient data.

65. An American university is reviewing the vaccination records of international students who have recently been admitted to their undergraduate programs. If the students do not meet all of the university's vaccination requirements, they are asked to obtain the appropriate vaccinations and to then acquire and submit the necessary documentation for approval before coming to campus. Which vaccination type, if missing on the student medical record, would be LEAST likely to represent a quantitative deficiency in vaccination status for this university?

   a. Varicella
   b. Measles, mumps, rubella (MMR)
   c. Human papillomavirus (HPV)
   d. Meningitis

66. A Health Information Management (HIM) Department specialist is running a report on patient insurance plans and the patients' corresponding places of work. This is done quarterly to assist with billing efficiency. Which of the following pieces of information would constitute a qualitative deficiency? (Assume that the date the report is run is 07-26-2019.)

   a. Daniel O. Lanoue/DOB 04-08-1956/O'Malley Attorneys at Law/Blue Cross Blue Shield
   b. Gladys R. Elliot/DOB 11-28-1947/Retired/Medicare
   c. Kristin D. Olsen/DOB 12-30-1988/Unemployed since 01-19-2019/COBRA
   d. Justin B. Horner/DOB 06-22-1975/Self-Employed Contractor/Ambetter (Health Insurance Marketplace)

67. Select the piece of patient data that represents a qualitative deficiency in the medical record. (Assume that the data are being pulled at a family physician's private practice.)

   a. "Blood Type: AB"
   b. "Allergies: N/A"
   c. "Diet Recommendations (newly diabetic): Fish-based Mediterranean"
   d. "Rx: Xanax (alprazolam), 15 mg daily"

68. The Centers for Disease Control and Prevention (CDC) performed an ongoing nationwide survey of deaths due to COVID-19 in 2020. Which of the following pieces of abstracted data would be LEAST useful to this survey request?

   a. Ethnicity/Race
   b. Underlying medical conditions
   c. Discharge status
   d. Admission source

69. A research hospital is partnering with a privately owned medical outreach program to determine the most urgent health needs of recent immigrant refugees from Myanmar. A data abstraction is performed after compiling their medical records. Which of the following data fields is LEAST likely to be abstracted for this purpose?

   a. Number of pregnancies
   b. Number of children with suspected rickets
   c. Number of malaria infections
   d. Number of cases of myopia

**70.** A retired secretary who just turned 65 years old consults a Medicare advisor to assist her with enrollment in Medicare Part D. Upon receipt of her application, the advisor notices that L-methylfolate is on her medications list, which he finds odd. He navigates to the manufacturer's page and, to his surprise, discovers that although it is considered a nutritional supplement, it can, in fact, be prescribed by a qualified healthcare professional. This is because it is known to boost the production of neurotransmitters in patients with a mutation that would otherwise keep production below normal. The advisor has never seen a case like this before and decides that he needs some clarification before initiating the patient's enrollment. Who would be the best person for the advisor to contact for more information about a "prescribed" supplement?

    a. The patient's primary care physician
    b. The patient's dietitian
    c. The patient's psychiatrist
    d. The patient's psychotherapist

**71.** An orthopedic surgeon is scheduled for a consultation with a 34-year-old patient in need of a hip replacement. The patient's hip weakness and pain arose as an (expected) consequence of rigorous chemotherapy and radiation for pediatric leukemia. Select the patient's electronic health record (EHR) to be requested that would NOT be necessary for the orthopedist's review prior to the consultation.

    a. Preoperative x-rays (radiology)
    b. Allergies to MAC anesthetics, if any (anesthesiology)
    c. Complete cancer treatment record (oncology)
    d. List of current medications (internal medicine)

**72.** Which of the following is UNTRUE about the enterprise-wide master patient index (EMPI)?

    a. It contains and connects unique patient healthcare vertical treatment/care paths.
    b. It includes software tools for flagging duplicate files.
    c. It effectively stores compliance policies and internal audit data.
    d. It maintains records of patient treatment/care for a 10-year minimum unless otherwise specified by the state.

**73.** According to the legislation enacted under HIPAA, what crucial piece of data theoretically BEST helps to avoid keeping several separate healthcare accounts for the same patient?

    a. A social security number
    b. A national patient identifier
    c. A Medicare policy number
    d. A national provider identifier

74. Select the statement that does NOT apply to provider education about writing notes for drugs administered in the HCPCS-II Drug Index.
    a. "If medication is given, be sure to specify how it was applied: was it topical? Inhaled? Ingested orally?"
    b. "Be sure to indicate the exact dosage of drugs and biologicals given to avoid any rejected claims."
    c. "*Always* report drugs administered in the outpatient setting, regardless of who provides you with them."
    d. "When in the emergency department, remember that the *facility* is responsible for reporting drug administration."

75. Select the statement that correctly applies to provider education about writing notes for vaccines administered in the "Medicine" section of the CPT codebook.
    a. "Do not counsel a patient and administer a vaccine during the same patient encounter; this is considered 'unbundling' by most payers."
    b. "If the reason for an office visit is strictly for receiving a vaccine, you may report both services separately."
    c. "Always remember that vaccine administration is *not* age dependent."
    d. "All vaccine administrations must document *both* the type and route of administration."

76. Which of the following data analysis reports is used primarily to generate reimbursement rates for beneficiaries enrolled in Medicare or Medicaid?
    a. Case mix index analysis
    b. Mortality rate analysis
    c. Inpatient coding accuracy analysis
    d. Average length of patient stay analysis

77. The first phase of clinical trials for a new chemotherapy drug is underway. Which of the following data analysis reports would prove MOST useful once concluded?
    a. Trends in Patient Cancer Treatment Histories
    b. Trends in Inpatient versus Outpatient Drug Treatments
    c. Trends in Adverse Reactions
    d. Trends in the Effects of Placebo Administration

78. Which of the following ICD-10 diagnosis codes is NOT consistent with the written documentation given?
    a. Laceration of popliteal artery, sequela; S85.019
    b. Fever NOS; R50.9
    c. Rosacea conjunctivitis, left eye; H10.822
    d. Fall from snow skis; V00.321

79. An employee at Medicare is reviewing the coding and documentation for an in-situ hybridization staining procedure performed on three specimens using fluorescence technology. Select the code set that correctly reflects this service.
    a. 88346-22
    b. 88346, 88350×3
    c. 88365, 88364-51
    d. 88365, 88364×2

80. Which of the following service codes is appended CORRECTLY with modifier 51?
    a. 20697-51
    b. 61107-51
    c. 11200-51
    d. 93612-51

81. Which of the following place-of-service codes is assigned INCORRECTLY?
    a. 02 – Dr. Morris, orthopedic ward – for telehealth follow-up with patient out of town
    b. 25 – Dr. Naff, OB-GYN – delivered healthy twin boys via cesarean section
    c. 12 – Dr. Erikson, intensive care unit – ongoing care of patients with severe cases of COVID-19
    d. 23 – Dr. Bootes, managing physician – pumped the stomach of a 19-year-old male with alcohol poisoning

82. A young, newly board-certified doctor presents to a temporary group living home for low-functioning adults as part of her office community service commitment. A patient with severe Down syndrome presents with his caretaker for a routine wellness check. It is a difficult visit as the patient, who is otherwise healthy, won't stop screaming, kicking, punching, and biting. The checkup, performed with difficulty, takes three times longer than anticipated, but it concludes with no abnormal findings. The exasperated doctor reports code 99345. What would a coder likely advise the doctor for the encounter?
    a. "This is technically a preventative medicine service—99387 would be the best option."
    b. "This looks good, but I'd append modifier 96 to this code as well."
    c. "Medicare will require additional documentation from me in order to use this code. Can you tell me about the visit in more detail?"
    d. "Medicare will not cover 99345 for this encounter."

83. A young doctor approaching the end of his residency status presents to the emergency department and is informed that his supervising physician is stuck in traffic due to a car wreck on the interstate and won't be in for another hour. The emergency department is already understaffed that day and is overwhelmed with patients. A small boy in need of sutures on his foot hasn't stopped screaming for an hour and is clearly agitating everyone present. The resident, who doesn't want to turn the boy away, gives him a local anesthetic, three small sutures, and then discharges him. The supervising physician later reports the physician-level service codes for the resident himself. How could this be problematic for a coder?
    a. The coder would need a letter from the resident's supervising physician to justify the physician-only codes reported.
    b. The coder could be equally liable for perpetuating fraudulent activity if he or she reported the physician-only service codes.
    c. The coder should tell the physician to report both codes separately if he wants to avoid an auditing investigation.
    d. The coder would be required by law to report the inappropriately documented claim to the supervising physician's board ethics committee.

84. A physician prescribes a new medication for a patient and writes that it is for "diabetic peripheral neuropathy." Which of the following queries would LEAST apply to what the coder needs?
    a. "Is the type of diabetes known?"
    b. "What is this patient's typical A1C range without medication?"
    c. "Is the diabetes a result of underlying disease?"
    d. "Was the diabetes induced due to drugs or chemicals?"

85. The notes for a procedure in the hospital radiology department indicate that an in-house radiologist and a technician were present when it was performed. During a phone call with the coder, the doctor first confirms that the radiology technologist was present. He noticed she was nervous because it was her first day, so as a courtesy, the doctor performed the procedure himself using the hospital's equipment before also providing the interpretation of results. The procedure in question was an MRI of the neck without contrast material. What is the correct code or sequence of codes?
    a. 70540
    b. 70540-TC-26
    c. 70540-26, 70540-TC
    d. 70540-22

86. What is the best online resource for researching the latest CPT coding changes?
    a. Office of the Inspector General (OIG)
    b. American Medical Association (AMA)
    c. Food and Drug Administration (FDA)
    d. Centers for Disease Control and Prevention (CDC)

87. Select the statement that is UNTRUE about the CPT coding update system.
    a. CPT category II codes become effective three months following their initial release.
    b. CPT category I codes appear in the updated codebook as early as the summer before their effective date, January 1.
    c. CPT Appendix B (Additions, Deletions, and Revisions) lists all code changes from the two previous years leading up to the current year.
    d. CPT category III codes are updated two times per year.

88. From the CMS website:

    2021 ICD-10-CM: COVID-19 UPDATE
    In response to the national emergency that was declared concerning the COVID-19 outbreak, the ... CDC['s] National Center for Health Statistics is implementing six new diagnosis codes into the ... ICD-10-CM, effective January 1, 2021.

Select the most appropriate resource from the list of downloads that gives a coder the MOST information about how to sequence COVID-19 codes.
    a. 2021 Code Tables, Tabular, and Index
    b. 20021 Conversion Table
    c. 2021 Code Descriptions in Tabular Order
    d. 2021 Coding Guidelines

89. The following data are taken from a CMS spreadsheet regarding the 2021 coding updates for COVID-19:

| CURRENT | EFFECTIVE | PREVIOUS |
|---------|-----------|----------|
| J12.82 | 1/1/2021 | J12.89 |
| M35.81 | 1/1/2021 | M35.8 |
| M35.89 | 1/1/2021 | M35.8 |
| Z11.52 | 1/1/2021 | Z11.59 |
| Z20.822 | 1/1/2021 | Z20.828 |
| Z86.16 | 1/1/2021 | Z86.19 |

If it is now March 2021, which of these code sequences would be appropriate for an immunocompromised patient who presents for a COVID-19 screening due to having already contracted the virus in the past, resulting in pneumonia? (Note: this encounter is purely precautionary due to the patient's weakened immune status since birth.)

   a. Z11.52, J12.82, D84.9
   b. Z11.52, Z20.822, M35.81
   c. Z11.52, Z86.16, J12.82
   d. Z11.52, Z86.16, D84.9

90. The following is taken from a PDF accessible online at cdc.gov with coding information that took effect in 2019:

> For patients documented with electronic cigarette (e-cigarette), or vaping, product use-associated lung injury, assign the code for the specific condition, such as

- J68.0, Bronchitis and pneumonitis due to chemicals, gases, fumes, and vapors; includes chemical pneumonitis
- J69.1, Pneumonitis due to inhalation of oils and essences; includes lipoid pneumonia
- J80, Acute respiratory distress syndrome
- J82, Pulmonary eosinophilia, not elsewhere classified
- J84.114, Acute interstitial pneumonitis
- J84.89, Other specified interstitial pulmonary disease.

A physician admits a patient with severe dyspnea and chest pain to the hospital. He suspects pulmonary eosinophilia. Later, he submits his initial report to the coder with a diagnosis of "pulmonary infiltrate NOS." Choose the best code(s) for the patient.

   a. R07.9, R06.00
   b. J82, R07.9, R06.00
   c. R91.8
   d. J82

91. The 2020 conversion factor (CF) for State X was $34.7701. For 2021, it has been adjusted to $35.0785. Calculate the 2021 facility pricing amount (FPA), Medicare payment (MP), State X, for CPT E/M code 99213, using the following information:

    E/M code 99213
    Work RVU: 0.95; FAC PE RVU: 0.39; MP RVU: 0.06
    Practice cost index: State X
    Work GPCI 1.000; PE GPCI 0.992; MP GPCI 1.088

**FPA = [(Work RVU) × (Work GPCI) + (FAC PE RVU) × (PE GPCI) + (MP RVU) × (MP GCPI)] × CF**

    a. $69.79
    b. $49.19
    c. $48.23
    d. $50.85

92. The 2020 conversion factor (CF) for State Y was $32.0551. For 2021, it has been adjusted to $32.1618. Calculate the 2021 non-facility pricing amount (NFPA), Medicare payment, State Y, for CPT E/M code 99214, using the following information:

    E/M Code 99214
    Work RVU: 0.92; NON-FAC PE RVU: 1.85;
    MP RVU: 0.07
    Practice Cost Index: State Y
    Work GPCI 1.500; PE GPCI 1.029;
    MP GPCI 0.791

**NFPA = [(Work RVU) × (Work GPCI) + (NON-FAC PE RVU) × (PE GPCI) + (MP RVU) × (MP GCPI)] × CF**

    a. $107.39
    b. $123.42
    c. $118.10
    d. $107.79

93. A young doctor who was recently board certified has just joined a practice. The in-house biller/coder is immediately tasked with helping her understand the discrepancies between the HIPAA 1995 and 1997 documentation guidelines for compliant E/M coding. Select the recommendation that correctly applies the basic principles of these guidelines.

    a. "Use medical necessity as a tool to select the guidelines that best characterize your individual patient encounters."
    b. "The 1995 guidelines are not open to interpretation; the 1997 guidelines have more gray areas. How you interpret those gray areas is your call."
    c. "The 1997 guidelines are not helpful with regard to note taking during an encounter; the 1995 guidelines are better suited for this purpose when first starting out."
    d. "We've found that carriers are relatively lenient with regard to what constitutes 'limited,' 'extended,' and 'complete' exams—just use your best judgment."

94. A coder/biller notices that one of his associates in the department is frequently miscoding patient hydration services. Select the suggestion that the coder/biller is LEAST LIKELY to make to this associate.
    a. "If a patient is given intravenous hydration overnight lasting into the next day, be sure to report the service continuously instead of separately."
    b. "Remember not to report a patient infusion as a hydration procedure if the patient is being administered drugs."
    c. "Make sure to add a modifier to the hydration code if it is administered by staff instead of the physician managing the patient."
    d. "If hydrating a patient before administering a chemotherapy infusion, be sure to do so for at least 31 minutes before switching."

95. Select the role that the internal compliance officer at a physician's practice does NOT play in preparation for an external audit.
    a. Provides guidance when drafting compliance plan additions, modifications, and deletions as needed within the workplace
    b. Serves as the point of contact for resolving any internal compliance violations
    c. Participates in the ongoing development of the OIGs Work Plan projects
    d. Spearheads all regular monitoring procedures to ensure successful implementation of the established compliance plan

96. A compliance officer is made aware of a policy violation. Depending on the nature and severity of the situation, which of the following corrective actions would NOT be taken by the officer?
    a. Immediately implementing the procedures outlined in a previously established corrective action plan
    b. Personally overseeing a partial refund to a patient who was egregiously overbilled
    c. Contacting the appropriate law enforcement agencies
    d. Consulting with an OIG lawyer in preparation for filing a potential lawsuit

97. As a general rule, which of the following components of the patient EHR best maintains the integrity of his or her healthcare record?
    a. Qualitative data
    b. Semantic data
    c. Quantitative data
    d. Validated data

98. What is an encoder?
    a. An automatic encryption tool for manually securing PHI data
    b. A person who assigns diagnostic and service codes to patient reports on a digital interface
    c. Software that facilitates proper code selection based on data autocollected in patient reports
    d. A digital version of a codebook, such as the ICD-10 or CPT, for quicker reference on a computer

**99. Select a vital feature of a practice management system that an IT/HIM department should consider when selecting one.**

a. Promotes quality patient care
b. User-friendly interface for writing patient reports
c. Contains a fully integrated EHR
d. Built-in physician calendar and scheduling management tools

**100. Select the pitfall of CAC coding software that has the MOST significant effect on autocoding accuracy and efficiency for patient reports over time.**

a. CAC-assigned codes must always be double-checked by coders.
b. The quality of a CAC's data input directly affects the quality of its data output.
c. The prevalence of CAC software risks putting coders out of work.
d. Artificial intelligence can make coding errors at a faster rate than a person.

**101. A doctor sees a patient who comes in feeling ill. After a thorough checkup, the doctor is unable to determine the cause of the patient's illness, and sends him a referral to the laboratory to run some tests. He lists the patient's symptoms on his patient report as follows: "1. Fever 2. Chills 3. Nausea 4. Vomiting." The brand-new CAC software analyzes the notes and assigns the following codes: R50.9, R68.83, R11.0, R11.10. A coder is proofing the CAC's work. What would be her BEST response to the software's autocoding choices?**

a. The codes rendered are all correct; they can be validated.
b. The four codes rendered are inaccurate; the coder should correct them using two codes (R50.9, R11.2) instead.
c. The four codes are inaccurate; the coder should correct them using three codes (R50.9, R68.83, R11.2) instead.
d. The coder should consult the physician for more information.

**102. Which of the following scenarios represents a breach of patient confidentiality under HIPAA?**

a. A psychiatrist schedules an appointment with a patient's father per the patient's request sent via email.
b. The boyfriend of a woman in a suicide ward calls the facility; they tell him they cannot confirm or deny her presence there.
c. An OB-GYN's nurse calls a patient's cell phone with her Pap test results and leaves a message, per the patient's contact preferences on file at the office.
d. A primary care physician, who has just accepted a new patient, has his nurse request the patient's medical records from his previous primary care physician.

**103. A human resources (HR) administrator in a hospital is giving a PowerPoint presentation for healthcare workers and providers regarding COVID-19 vaccine status and HIPAA rights. Based on your knowledge of HIPAA, which of the following presentation titles would NOT apply to this issue?**

a. "Vaccine 'Status' Passports: An Up-and-Coming Trend in Travel"
b. "Why Asking 'Are You Vaccinated?' Is Not a Violation of HIPAA Rights"
c. "Maintaining Patient Integrity: A Step-by-Step Guide to Sharing Vaccination Records to COVID-19-Conscious Employers"
d. "'Don't Mask, Don't Tell': The Legal Ramifications for Patients Who Falsify Their COVID-19 Vaccine Status"

104. A 19-year-old Lebanese patient who lives with her bilingual older sister walks into a Planned Parenthood clinic on a Saturday in New York City to discuss the results of her sexually transmitted disease testing. She understands English better than she can speak it, so an interpreter had been scheduled in advance for her follow-up. Unfortunately, the interpreter cancels at the last minute and another one won't be available until later the next week. The clinic is very busy, and the nurse receptionist must act quickly. Select the scenario that would be considered a violation of the patient's privacy rights. (Note: the patient has no HIPAA release forms on file.)
   a. The nurse receptionist helps the patient reschedule her appointment with the help of a 24-hour phone interpreter.
   b. The nurse receptionist calls the home phone number on file for the patient to check whether her sister can come interpret for her today.
   c. A bilingual patient from Syria, also in the waiting area, offers to help the nurse explain to the patient why she can't be seen (i.e., the interpreter isn't coming).
   d. After rescheduling the appointment, the patient is sent home with an educational pamphlet in Arabic about sexually transmitted diseases.

105. During the COVID-19 pandemic, a medical assistant spends every other weekday scheduling patients to see their doctors at home for virtual visits. She is given a laptop to use in both her work and home environments. She signs a special security agreement in order to do so. Which of the following would NOT apply to such an agreement to maintain maximum security of sensitive (including HIPAA-protected) information?
   a. Regularly running and maintaining antivirus software
   b. Keeping all sensitive documents on the laptop's hard drive encryption software
   c. Using a USB thumb drive to access her home files for personal use
   d. Changing her laptop login password every month using an autogenerator

106. Which one of the following recommended elements of a password is LEAST effective in maintaining the security of a medical database system?
   a. Special characters (@, !, *, etc.)
   b. A number series entered in increasing order (1, 2, 3, etc.)
   c. A mix of upper- and lowercase letters (a, U, t, Y, etc.)
   d. The use of underscores between characters

107. Administrators at ACME, Inc. Medical Research are compiling all cancer lab reports in the United States from the past 20 years for a study directed by the nation's top oncologists. Which piece of information on a lab report would represent a violation of the minimum necessary standard instituted by HIPAA?
   a. The complete results of a pathology study on a patient
   b. The full name and address of the patient's referring physician
   c. The laboratory CLIA number
   d. The patient's hospital ID number

108. A patient signed a HIPAA release form in the office today. Select the HR department to which it should be submitted for authorization approval.
   a. EHR
   b. HIM
   c. IGPHC
   d. HIT

**109. What kind of patient data in any healthcare setting MUST be protected through digital encryption?**
   a. PHI
   b. Employment/insurance history
   c. Sociodemographic data
   d. Current age and sex/gender

**110. Which of the following methods of data transfer would not meet health information exchange standards?**
   a. Operating through an https:// online platform
   b. Requiring email recipients to use the sender's digital ID for access to messages
   c. Portals secured through verified digital certificates
   d. Sharing cloud-encrypted data through an open link to the recipient

**111. Select the confidential record-keeping strategy that is LEAST appropriate in a healthcare setting.**
   a. Retaining all paper patient records locked in index-based filing cabinets
   b. Leaving a social security number on a Post-it Note for reference while working on patient claims
   c. Digital encryption of all registered patient PHI
   d. Backing up all confidential records using secure cloud-based software

**112. Select the BEST way to appropriately destroy confidential patient records.**
   a. Emptying the desktop recycle bin
   b. Hiring a shredding company
   c. Shredding in house before taking papers to the dumpster
   d. Deleting a patient's profile from the office client management software

# Answer Key and Explanations for Test #1

**1. C:** This is a relatively common diagnosis. If both symptoms are unspecified and occurring together, they are coded with a combination code. This means that coding R11.0 and R11.10 together would be inappropriate. Additionally, the individual codes R11.0 (nausea, not otherwise specified [NOS]) and R11.10 (vomiting, unspecified) are clearly not combination codes because they are mutually exclusive. Therefore, the use of either one is insufficient to appropriately document the patient's complaint. The correct combination diagnosis code is R11.2, nausea with vomiting, unspecified.

**2. B:** To find the correct diagnosis, turn to the Table of Neoplasms in the ICD-10. Under the category "Breast," there is a subcategory of "Upper-inner quadrant." Because this neoplasm is specified as being malignant, using the base code indicated in the table, C50.2-, would be the first step to identifying the exact numeric code. The patient is designated as male, which eliminates C50.211 and C50.411. The correct answer is C50.221, because the cancer is in his right breast and in the upper-inner quadrant (versus being in his left breast and in the upper-outer quadrant, as described by C50.421).

**3. D:** This patient's surgery involves a pacemaker upgrade. Because a pacemaker is not the same as a defibrillator, we can immediately eliminate 33249 with 33225 and 33241. This leaves us with 33228 or 33214. Upon closer examination, we can eliminate 33228 because the procedure is a removal and replacement of parts for an existing dual-lead system; i.e., the pacemaker system *remains the same before and after the procedure*. Therefore, 33214 is the correct answer. The entire purpose of the procedure is to *change the pacemaker system*. It not only explicitly mentions the implementation of a pacemaker "upgrade," but it also specifies that the upgrade involves a conversion of a "single-chamber" system to a "dual-chamber" system.

**4. A:** In medicine, PHI is the acronym for protected health information. Private, personal, and patient are some of the individual components of PHI. However, what matters most in the modern healthcare infrastructure (which has largely become information technology [IT] dependent) is the fact that this information is meant to be kept confidential across digital systems and interfaces. It is therefore protected by law under the Health Insurance Portability and Accountability Act of 1996 (HIPAA), and any electronic sharing of PHI must comply with the "minimum necessary" standard in order to maximize patient privacy and confidentiality.

**5. B:** Medicare is federally funded ONLY and exclusively for seniors 65 and older. Medicaid, however, is funded *both* federally and by the state in which the patient(s) live(s). It assists people of all ages with health insurance payment assistance and is a service used especially commonly by low-income and underprivileged individuals and families in the United States.

**6. B:** HIPAA and the Merit-Based Incentive Payment System (MIPS) are not forms. CMS-1450 (or UB-04) is a standard billing form that is used to submit patient claims to Medicare administrative contractors for services or procedures that inherently meet the "medically necessary" requirement for reimbursement. Because an Advance Beneficiary Notice of Non-Coverage (ABN) is completed when a service or procedure may *not* meet this "medically necessary" requirement, ABN is the correct answer.

**7. B:** The term "bilateral" indicates that the operation is being performed on a pair of body parts. This eliminates repair of uterus and removal of uterus because a woman normally only has one uterus. However, the prefix "salping-" means fallopian tube (versus the prefix "hyster-" for uterus).

The suffix "-ectomy" indicates that parts are being removed from the body, so removal of the fallopian tubes is the correct answer. If the patient were undergoing surgical repair of her fallopian tubes, the suffix would be "-rrhaphy" instead of "ectomy."

**8. D:** The acronym SOAP (which stands for subjective, objective, assessment, plan) is commonly used in the medical field. It represents all four crucial components of a physician's clinical documentation for the proper identification and management of a patient's medical issues. Prescription information is not a main pillar of the SOAP notes. Rather, it would be found (if at all) as a subcategory of the physician's treatment plan for the patient.

**9. D:** In obstetrics, the status G#P# is an acronym for the Latin terms gravida and para. Gravida indicates a given patient's number of previous pregnancies, and para indicates her number of previous deliveries that reached at least 20 weeks gestation.

**10. C:** The Office of the Inspector General (OIG) is not a coding manual, so OIG is easily eliminated. The ICD-10-CM is used primarily for coding diagnoses. The CPT is mostly used for coding services and procedures. The Healthcare Common Procedure Coding System Level II (HCPCS-II), however, contains codes for ordering various medical supplies, such as orthotics. Therefore, HCPCS-II is the correct answer.

**11. A:** Category Z is the correct answer because it contains the subindexes needed for coding routine patient care visits (including other details such as the patient's age group and "with" or "without abnormal findings"). The other categories listed are reserved for patients presenting with medical complaints; therefore, they require the appropriate diagnosis codes based on the physician's documentation. Category A is for "Certain infectious and parasitic diseases," and category K is for "Diseases of the digestive system." Category R is for "Symptoms, signs, and abnormal clinical and laboratory findings, not elsewhere classified," and it is often what coders turn to when a patient presents with symptoms, but his or her diagnosis cannot be determined at that time.

**12. D:** Category III codes are reserved exclusively for new and emerging technologies in medicine that are still being actively studied for their effectiveness and safety, so they haven't yet had the Food and Drug Administration (FDA) sign off its approval for widespread use as a category I code. Vascular imaging, although incredibly complex at times, is a standard sub-practice of the radiological field, so a category III code is unnecessary and inappropriate. Appendix A, in which indexes of modifiers can be found, is in no way directly related to the coding of procedures involving vascular systems (but it could be indirectly related, depending on whether or not the procedure itself requires flagging for special circumstances). Appendix C, although informative, covers complex cases in evaluation and management (E/M) coding only, so it would be irrelevant to the coder's needs. A highly skilled coder understands, however, that code selection and code sequencing for vascular imaging are highly dependent on the names and classifications of the vessels explored within the same session. Attention to detail here is therefore paramount. Appendix L is the answer.

**13. B:** When it comes to E/M code selection, this is a special circumstance in which the location of the patient's treatment (the hospital) trumps who treated the patient (his personal physician). With that information, office or outpatient services is automatically ruled out because in-hospital treatment is considered inpatient and because the physician in question is not seeing his patient at his own office (as an outpatient). Because the patient was not explicitly designated as being under observation status, this rules out initial observation care. The correct answer is subsequent hospital care because the initial hospital care E/M service guidelines explicitly state that these codes "are used to report the first hospital inpatient encounter with the patient by the admitting physician [AI]" (CPT 16). Because this is clearly not applicable to the second day of Mr. Greenbriar's treatment, the E/M series subsequent hospital care should be consulted for the appropriate E/M code.

**14. A:** Unless a coder is already familiar with emergency service guidelines, it is always recommended to read the guidelines first because there is often overlap into other categories depending on the case being examined. The codes 99283 and 99285, or codes categorized as emergency department services, can be immediately eliminated from the list due to a crucial guideline found in this series of codes: "[f]or critical care services provided in the emergency department, see critical care notes and 99291, 99292." Upon consultation of the critical care notes and codes, it is made clear that code assignment for this particular patient is entirely dependent on the duration of care received "on a given date." Further, the table "Total Duration of Critical Care Codes" indicates that time spent with a patient spanning anywhere from 105 to 134 minutes is coded as 99291 and 99292×2, which is the correct coding set and sequence because it is stated that the physician spent 105 total minutes with the patient that day. This eliminates the second set of codes from the choice list: 99291, 99292.

**15. A:** The answer to this question is easily gleaned from a careful reading of the hospital discharge services guidelines. The statement regarding code 99239 is untrue because it is written that final examinations of the patient are performed "as appropriate" for either 99238 or 99239, and it is therefore not limited to one or the other. The statement regarding nursing facility care is untrue because a parenthetical note near the end of the "Hospital discharge services" section reads "For nursing facility care discharge, see 99315, 99316." The statement about a 30-minute discharge is untrue because code 99239 (versus its counterpart, 99238) specifically indicates that it is used only for "Hospital discharge day management" of "more than 30 minutes." So a discharge timed at exactly 30 minutes would be coded with 99238 instead. The first statement addressing same-day admission and discharge is true because the guidelines stipulate that "[f]or a patient admitted and discharged from ... inpatient status on the same date, the services should be reported with codes 99234–99236 as appropriate." Therefore, the only true statement in this choice list addresses same-day admission/discharge.

**16. D:** Chief complaint, history of present illness, and review of systems are subcategories of the first pillar of E/M services—history. During this first stage of evaluation, the physician reviews or gathers basic data about the patient's reason for the visit. By contrast, level of risk is a subcategory of the last pillar, medical decision making, and it is consequently one of the last pieces of data reviewed with the patient, if at all. This is because the idea of "risk" usually implies a direct relationship between the patient's current health status and the health risks potentially incurred through a treatment option involving surgery.

**17. D:** When a physician has officially accepted responsibility for a patient's care after a consultation appointment by referral, this constitutes what is known as an official transfer of care (i.e., from one physician to another). When this happens at the conclusion of an initial consultation appointment, the coder is instructed to "use the appropriate office or other outpatient consultation codes and then the established patient office or other outpatient services codes" (CPT 19). Because this is Kendra's second visit with Dr. Yakamoto after being accepted as a new patient in his office last week, this automatically rules out codes 99243 and 99254 because these are both consultation codes so they are no longer applicable to Kendra. The code 99203 is used for new patients only, and the aforementioned guidelines advise against this choice. Therefore, 99213, an office code for an established patient, is the correct answer.

**18. B:** In the CPT codebook, it is important to differentiate between E/M code sets that are for patients presenting to the office with a medical complaint versus patients who are presenting for a routine preventative medicine checkup. Because the boy is healthy and presents without complaint to his appointment (likely an annual visit), 99201 and 99211 can be eliminated from the list of choices. The codes 99393 and 99383 are specifically used for preventative medicine, and they are organized by patient age groups as well as whether or not it is a new or established patient. Because both codes account for the boy's age correctly (5–11 years of age), the correct choice can be determined through the patient's record with the doctor. Because it is implied that the child has seen this pediatrician before, 99383 is ruled out. The correct answer is 99393.

**19. C:** In anesthesiology services, modifiers are crucial for proper reimbursement because the entity covering the service will adjust pay based on who performed the service. In this case, an anesthesia resident was performing services needed under the direct guidance and supervision of the anesthesiologist. Therefore, modifier GC would document the nature of these services correctly. This eliminates both answers that include modifier QY in the final code sequence because modifier QY is used when a certified registered nurse anesthetist is performing services under the medical direction of the anesthesiologist (versus a resident). Finally, modifier sequence P1-GC-QS is incorrect because the patient health status (P1) always appears at the end of an anesthesiology modifier sequence, preceded by QS (MAC services, if applicable), which is further preceded by who performed the procedure, GC in this case. It would make sense, then, that the anesthesiologist would tell this new coder to simply replace modifier QY with modifier GC for a total modifier sequence of GC-QS-P1.

**20. C:** Modifiers 76 and 77 are defined as repeat procedure(s) or service(s), whether by the same or a different surgeon. This is not a repeat attempt at the medullary implant procedure; rather, it is a procedure that is targeted at mitigating the complications incurred from the first procedure. Because the reaction is specified as being rare, it can be safely assumed that this second operation was unexpected. This second procedure was performed by the same surgeon who performed the first, Dr. Rigo. Modifier 78 fits this description, defined as an unplanned return to the operating/procedure room by the same surgeon. The use of modifier 79 is ruled out because it only flags unrelated procedures within the global surgical package period; therefore, modifier 78 is the correct answer.

**21. C:** A surgeon who discontinues a procedure is a relatively common occurrence across most disciplines in surgical medicine. A useful strategy to use as a coder when this happens is to try to understand coding protocol through the lens of the Centers for Medicare & Medicaid Services (CMS)—whether through a medical necessity perspective, a financial one, or both. To start, not reporting the incision and drainage procedure at all doesn't make logical sense from either perspective. Why would CMS cover a lidocaine injection alone without further documentation of its necessity? The procedure must be included in the claim for this purpose; however, it must also be appended with a modifier as a flag for special circumstances that CMS should consider. Modifiers 52 and 53 are easy to confuse with one another, but a discontinued procedure (modifier 53) is not synonymous with reduced services (modifier 52) in coding. A great way to differentiate between them is to remember that modifier 52 assumes that the procedure was completed in full; modifier 53 does not. Therefore, because the incision and drainage procedure was attempted but discontinued due to the physician's concern for the patient's well-being and safety, reporting it with modifier 53 is the most appropriate answer.

**22. B:** The patient is presenting to the hospital for the first time during this particular encounter. This eliminates 99233, a code for subsequent hospital care, implying that the patient has been in the hospital for at least 24 hours. It also eliminates 99236, an observation services code, which is not applicable to this patient's initial intake at the hospital. For the initial hospital care codes 99222 and 99223, the distinction between the level of E/M services rendered is fairly clear. Although both codes require a history and exam that are comprehensive, only 99223 requires that medical decision making be the highest in complexity (compared to code 99222 requires only moderate complexity). The code 99223 is appropriate for this encounter.

**23. B:** Although it is true that Dr. Arapoglou is explicitly present and on standby during the delivery, the delivery took only 10 minutes before he went to work on resuscitating the newborn. This means that code 99360, "standby service for a high-risk delivery," is not reported because its use requires that the physician on standby be present for 30 minutes or more (versus the 10 that were documented). Consequently, this means that the code pair 99465, 99360 is also not reported. The code 99465 itself is of interest, however, because it is the code for basic delivery/birthing room resuscitation services for newborns in cardiopulmonary distress. This description is consistent with the report. The parenthetical notes under code 99465 further indicate that it can be paired with other codes as necessary; however, code 99464 is not one of them: "Do not report 99465 in conjunction with 99464." Therefore, the only code needed to report Dr. Arapoglou's services for this encounter is 99465.

**24. C:** Although there is constant oversight of potentially unstable psychiatric patients in this facility, it still doesn't constitute observation status, so 99220 is incorrect. Additionally, 99223 is an initial hospital care code, which seems like it would be appropriate upon first glance; however, codes pertaining to "a patient in a psychiatric residential treatment center" are to be taken from the nursing facility services E/M category, so 99223 no longer applies. The codes 99306 and 99310 are both listed in this same category; but, upon further scrutiny, code 99310 is reserved for subsequent nursing facility patient encounters only. This means that 99306, which specifically applies to a patient's initial encounter for admission to such a facility, is the correct answer.

**25. A:** Because the patient is visiting a facility open to anyone who needs immediate medical attention in a nonemergency situation, it is safe to assume that the patient is not established by this particular physician during her visit. This easily eliminates codes 99213 and 99215. The remaining two codes in the "New patient" subsection, 99201 and 99202, require strict adherence to their individual E/M requirements in order to be reported. Code 99201, for example, requires these three key components: a problem-focused history, a problem-focused examination, and straightforward medical decision making. The documentation states that the patient's history and exam were of an expanded problem-focused nature. Therefore, this code cannot be reported. By contrast, code 99202, although it also requires straightforward medical decision making, also requires that the care be centered around expanded approaches to the patient's history and exam. Code 99202 is the proper code for this encounter.

**26. A:** The pediatrician's documentation suggests that Sofia has presented for her second annual checkup, and, overall, she appears to be very healthy for her age. Therefore, the best place to look for coding her visit would be found in the "Preventative medicine" subsection of the CPT E/M Guideline Chapter. Codes 99201 and 99211 are office or other outpatient codes, which don't apply to this encounter because Sofia presents without complaint and is simply having her routine annual checkup. Because it is also implied that she is an established patient, the only appropriate answer would be 99393 (versus the new-patient code for the same age range, 99383).

**27. D:** Code 99385 does not apply to Dan's situation because codes in the preventative medicine subcategory of E/M services are used in routine health checkups for patients without medical complaints. Dan presents to the new specialist with a health concern despite being healthy, so his case is not applicable here. Codes 99408 and 99409 are for behavior change interventions, and they both specifically address the issue of alcoholism, which makes them tempting choices. However, a careful reading of the guidelines in the "Counseling risk factor reduction and behavior change intervention" section states that "Behavior change interventions are for persons who have a behavior that is often considered an illness itself, such as ... substance abuse/misuse[.]" Codes 99408 and 99409 are therefore problematic. Dan may be a self-described heavy drinker, but, per his clean health record, he is not a known alcoholic from a clinical standpoint. Further, he has no health issues other than the behavior he wishes to change now that he knows he's genetically prone to liver disease. This is key, because the same guidelines mentioned above also stipulate that "risk factor reduction interventions... should address such issues as... substance use... and diagnostic and laboratory test results available at the time of the encounter." Such services are also reported "for persons without a specific illness for which the counseling might otherwise be used as part of treatment." This means that 99402 is the correct code for this encounter.

**28. C:** Code 32097 is incorrect because it only documents the initial procedure, "thoracotomy, with diagnostic biopsy(ies) of lung nodule(s)... unilateral." Code 32098 is also incorrect because it documents a completely different initial procedure, which includes a thoracotomy, but only biopsies the pleural space. Code 32120, by contrast, addresses the surgical nature of the second procedure because it is performed for postoperative complications related to the previous procedure. Selecting the appropriate modifier comes down to the coder's attention to detail: because the documentation states that the surgeon "perform[ed] a repeat thoracotomy," the use of 32120-76 appears at first to be the correct choice. A seasoned coder, however, knows that the context in which this repeat thoracotomy procedure was performed will most affect the choice of modifier beyond the simple use of this term alone. To illustrate, the first thoracotomy was made to perform a biopsy; the second was made to control a postoperative emergency of severe internal bleeding. This was clearly not a repeat procedure for a biopsy. The surgeon may have made use of the previous site of incision, but only in order to access and remedy the hemorrhaging tissue. Code 32120-78 appropriately documents an unexpected complication involving a return to the operating room with the same surgeon who performed the initial procedure.

**29. B:** Surgery involving eyelids can be complicated from a coding perspective because the type of surgery performed will determine which section of codes to consult. First of all, it is explicitly stated that the nature of the injury, as well as the surgery Dr. Tardy is performing, involves skin only and requires an intermediate level of repair. This means that we can bypass the 60000-level surgery codes. Indeed, under the subsection here entitled "Reconstruction," there is a parenthetical reference that states "For repair of skin of eyelid, see 12011-12018, 12051-12057, 13151-13153." This means that, even without regard for modifiers, 67930-22-E3-E4 and 67930-E3-E4, 67938 are not applicable. Code 12051, along with code 12052, are "intermediate" repair codes for the skin on the eyelids; unfortunately, code 12051 only allows for up to 2.5 cm of repairs to be eligible for reporting. Code 12052, in contrast, can be reported for any injury repair between 2.6 and 5.0 cm in length. Because Dr. Tardy documented 2.8 cm of total skin repair, code 12052 is the best choice. Modifiers are also needed to most accurately document the difficulty and locale of the surgery itself. Adding modifier 22, "Increased procedural services," indicates that extra work was required beyond the normal parameters of surgery (in this case, an "unusual amount of flushing and cleaning for 20 extra minutes"). The HCPCS-II E3 and E4 modifiers indicate that the surgery was performed on the right upper and lower eyelids, respectively. Finally, because modifier 22 most affects how the procedure is reimbursed, it is sequenced first.

**30. B:** This is a tricky situation in which two completely unrelated services are rendered during the same E/M visit. Code 99212 alone would have been sufficient for an uneventful follow-up appointment with regard to the wart removal. Because a UTI test via urinalysis is a medical complaint that is unrelated to the reason for the patient's visit that day, but nonetheless deserves the physician's attention, CMS regulations require two codes. Code 99212×2 would also be inappropriate. This is because the doctor needs to be reimbursed for two separate E/M services that happened to warrant attention in just one visit, and CMS will look for information that justifies the payments for both. This is done with modifiers. 99212, 99212-59, with -59 flagging the encounter as requiring an unexpected but "Distinct procedural service," is closer to what CMS needs; however, it isn't the best choice here because modifier 59 would be more appropriate for non-E/M services and procedures. Code 99212, 99212-25, however, is the best choice. Unlike modifier 59, modifier 25 is specifically used for E/M services only. It serves as a "flag" for a "Separately identifiable E/M service by the same physician" during the same visit. More importantly, it justifies the UTI test, which, for CMS, would not be considered a medical necessity during a follow-up for wart removal. Without modifier 25, the claim for the urinalysis would be denied and the physician wouldn't be paid for having it done.

**31. C:** Pain is easy to code incorrectly because the rules governing sequencing are rather complex. According to ICD-10 guidelines, if the reason for a patient's visit is specifically for pain treatment and/or management, then the G code is always sequenced first. This eliminates M54.40, G89.11, and M51.26, G89.11. Additionally, using G89.11 with M54.5, the code for low-back pain (lumbago,) is not the best option here because it is still possible to code for something much more specific. This can be gleaned from the EXCLUDES 1 Note under M54.5, indicating that "lumbago due to intervertebral disc displacement" is reported with M51.2-. Upon consultation of this section, code M51.26 codes for "other intervertebral disc displacement, lumbar region." Therefore, G89.11, M51.26 is the correct answer.

**32. A:** Because it is explicitly stated that Carlos is presenting for routine lab tests outside of his physician's office, it is automatically implied that there were no abnormal findings (i.e., medical issues of immediate concern) during his checkup earlier that day. This helps eliminate the use of code Z00.01. Along with his general health panel (80050), Carlos is having a basic metabolic panel performed; 80047 and 80048 code for basic metabolic, but 80053 codes for comprehensive metabolic. This means that sequence Z00.00, 80053, 80050 is incorrect. The correct sequence is Z00.00, 80047, 80050.

**33. D:** Gertrude's physician has sent her to an audiology center to either confirm or rule out his suspicion that she has developed a sudden onset of Ménière's disease. This means that any codes pertaining to Ménière's can be ruled out, because the diagnosis is only suspected—it is not certain. Therefore, H81.02 (Ménière's of the left ear) with 92257 or 92257-52 are not applicable to Gertrude. Code H91.22 is defined as "sudden idiopathic hearing loss, left ear" and is therefore a more accurate designation for Gertrude's current complaint. Code 92257 is correct for a comprehensive audiometry evaluation. The coder should have already noted, however, that Gertrude's hearing issues pertain only to one ear, her left, meaning that modifiers pertaining to laterality may be applicable. A careful review of the "Audiologic function tests" guidelines in the "Medicine" section of the CPT reveals an indication to "use modifier 52 if a test is applied to one ear instead of two ears." The correct answer, then, is H91.22, R42 (vertigo NOS), 92557-52.

**34. B:** Kaposi's sarcoma is an HIV-related illness. Because the patient is specified as having known HIV, a Kaposi's sarcoma implies that the patient is symptomatic (i.e., has AIDS), which eliminates the use of Z21 (an HIV-positive but asymptomatic patient). Otitis media is an ear infection with no known association to HIV. However, the infection is in both ears (bilateral), which eliminates all uses of H66.90 because ear laterality is unspecified. Therefore B20, C46.52, and H66.93 are all correct. Finally, in this instance, because being HIV-positive directly impacts the patient's care, the diagnosis of B20 (human immunodeficiency virus [HIV] disease) is sequenced first. It is then followed by the condition known to be directly associated with it (Kaposi's sarcoma) before any other unrelated condition, if applicable (in this case, bilateral otitis media).

**35. D:** Procedure codes 47563 and 47564 are not applicable because they include additional sub procedures that are not mentioned (cholecystectomy with cholangiography, cholecystectomy with exploration of common duct). It is also made clear that the anesthesiologist did not personally supervise the anesthesia procedure (AD) because he performed the anesthesia himself (AA). Therefore, the correct sequence of codes is 00790-AA-P1; 47562.

**36. D:** On January 1, 1998, CMS introduced a coding regulation requiring the use of G0105 or G0121 in lieu of 45378 for colonoscopy procedures performed as part of colorectal cancer screening in outpatient settings because CMS requires differentiation between those Medicare patients who are at a low or high risk for developing such a cancer (G0121 and G0105, respectively, which are both HCPCS-II codes). Therefore, because the standard CPT code 45378 would be denied (with or without modifiers), and Mr. Jeong is considered to have a low risk at the time of the procedure, G0121 is the correct code for this encounter.

**37. C:** Although CMS tends to prefer HCPCS-II G codes for outpatient colorectal cancer screenings, an exception can be made to this general rule when there are abnormal findings during the encounter. This does NOT mean, however, that G codes are to be used with CPT codes for such encounters. This, then, eliminates G0105, 45380. We also know that because George is a high-risk patient, G0121 is not applicable here either. CPT code 45378 is for a flexible diagnostic colonoscopy, and 45380 is the code for single or multiple biopsies during the same procedure. Because a parenthetical note clearly states not to use 45380 with 45378, 45380 is the best code for George. In general, whenever a diagnostic CPT procedure becomes a therapeutic CPT procedure, the diagnostic procedure is not reported because it is bundled into the overall surgical package for the encounter.

**38. B:** According to the ICD-10 CM/PCS MS-DRG Definitions Manual v38.1, alpha thalassemia is classified as a red blood cell disorder. Because it is not listed as a major hematological and immunological or coagulation disorder, this automatically eliminates 808 and 813. The classification table for red blood cell disorder clearly shows that when alpha thalassemia is also a major (secondary) complication or comorbidity, the appropriate DRG code is 811 (rather than 812, which is used when the condition exists but doesn't meet that particular criterion).

**39. D:** According to the ICD-10 CM/PCS MS-DRG Definitions Manual v38.1, diagnosis code 0VB07ZZ, or excision of prostate, via natural or artificial opening (in this case, the urethra, a natural opening) is classified as a transurethral prostatectomy-type procedure. This eliminates 707 and 708 because they are used in other major male pelvic procedures. The classification table for the diagnosis code in question includes 713 and 714 as the DRG codes with or without primary or secondary complication or comorbidity; therefore, the correct DRG code is 714.

**40. B:** APC codes are used by Medicare as a means for calculating reimbursements for varying categories of procedures. If multiple procedures and their respective APC codes are submitted to Medicare, only the APC code that indicates the highest rate of reimbursement will be applied to the payment made. This does not mean, however, that only one APC (the highest paying) should be reported without its lower paying counterpart. All applicable CPT codes in this case are therefore reported with all of their corresponding APC categories whether they are separately classified or not. Under no circumstances should the CPT codes in this particular case omit their respective APC codes, and vice versa. Such omitted information could have potential ramifications if discovered during an audit. Should a clear lack of transparency be discovered, an auditor may suspect the use of unethical coding approaches.

**41. C:** Status level indicator C for inpatient procedures is an APC code marker exclusively reserved for hospital outpatient centers, which is why it is unique to them only. It indicates the use of various medical supplies such as drugs, medical equipment, and procedural tools used for inpatient surgeries. These "C" items are specially covered by Medicare in addition to the procedures themselves through the Outpatient Prospective Payment System.

**42. B:** The National Correct Coding Initiative (NCCI) is a CMS regulation that demonstrates and implements ethical coding methodologies that aim to prevent reporting and reimbursement errors and/or fraud. It also helps clarify gray areas with regard to what is or is not included within certain global surgical packages. The two codes appearing in the first two columns on the left side of the table of edits indicate coding pairs identified and edited (in other words, flagged or labeled), mostly with a 1 or a 0. A 0 flags pairs of codes that cannot be reported together under any circumstances. Conversely, a 1 indicates pairs that can be used together, but only with the appropriate modifier(s), and under very specific circumstances. These circumstances (or lack thereof) are defined briefly in the last column on the right, which is also known as the procedure-to-procedure edit rationale. Therefore, the need for code pairs in the various existing tables (updated regularly) is characterized primarily by whether it is appropriate to use them together or not.

**43. C:** In the NCCI edits, the CCM indicator 1 designates a pair of codes that aren't normally reported together, but that may be in certain circumstances by appending the appropriate modifier. Denise can report codes 12345 and 54321 as long as they are sequenced and modified appropriately. Depending on the complexity of the situation, Denise might also consider adding a brief written report to her claim that clarifies the unique needs of the patient in question, making both services rendered medical necessary, albeit under unusual circumstances.

**44. A:** The choices regarding modifier 51 and the use of two add-on codes are easily ruled out first because, true or untrue, they don't apply to NCCI editing parameters, so they are irrelevant. Code 27889 is for a procedure known as ankle disarticulation, which is an amputation. Unlike most surgeries in orthopedics requiring intricate repairs, this procedure tends to be performed on the macroscopic level rather than on the microscopic level by its very nature. Therefore, codes 27889 and 69990 are also not inherently mutually exclusive, per se, because the use of an operating microscope is a fairly standard medical practice in orthopedic surgery. In this case, however, because the amputation procedure likely requires nothing more than visualization with magnifying loupes or corrected vision (per 69990 guidelines), an operating microscope isn't needed and is therefore (medically) unnecessary.

**45. D:** T codes are known as category III codes, which means that they represent new and emerging techniques and technologies that may or may not earn future FDA approval. If they do, they become category I codes and are thus considered standard medical practice. Although they are CMS-approved for use with some category I codes in some circumstances, there are other circumstances in which CMS would deem their use together as inappropriate. This is one such case, given the 0 NCCI edit designation; that is, codes 0230T and 11042 are NEVER to be reported together. If they are, CMS would deny the claim. The coder would also probably tell the doctor to use an alternative (but standard) numbing technique instead, just to ensure that he is reimbursed in full for all aspects of his work.

**46. A:** The patient presents with a medical complaint that is unusual for her history and therefore has an unknown underlying etiology. Because tachycardia can have a wide range of etiologies, both benign and disease-related, CMS would deem the electrocardiogram a medical necessity.

Generally, if a patient is alert and mobile at the time of a 911 call, an ambulance is not medically necessary. If her son found her on the kitchen floor unconscious after hearing her fall, an ambulance transport would be deemed medically necessary.

Astigmatism is a common diagnosis for blurred vision. This is generally corrected through the use of contacts and eyeglasses. Therefore, CMS would deem the laser vision correction surgery to be medically unnecessary because the astigmatism can be easily corrected through less invasive (and less expensive) means.

Performing a punch biopsy for acne is not an appropriate and justifiable service for addressing this patient's medical issue. The claim would be denied because the dermatologist did not first attempt to resolve the problem through simpler and less invasive means, such as recommending a readily available face wash from the drugstore or writing the patient a prescription.

**47. D:** Although it is true that CMS is the umbrella organization under which all national healthcare regulations are made, all regions of the United States nonetheless have some freedom to use or modify some regulations in order to best meet the needs of the populations that they serve. Thus, each region operates according to their own LCDs. If a service or procedure is listed as "retired" in the online LCD index, it means that the LCD had determined after a time that it would no longer be deemed "medically necessary" and would therefore no longer be covered in that region's Medicare services. Consequently, Mr. Johnson will likely be offered alternative forms of therapy that Medicare will cover.

**48. B:** NPI is the acronym for National Provider Identifier, a 10-digit number that a healthcare provider is required to have by HIPAA. Other entities that require this number include health insurance companies and healthcare clearinghouses. The use of this identifier is standard claim filing protocol because it is required by law.

**49. D:** A simplified claims submission process generally first involves the coder and/or biller making the appropriate code assignments based on the doctor's documentation of the patient encounter. This information is then entered electronically into a billing software system, along with other pertinent patient information, such as their demographics and health plan information. An e-claim is directly sent to a clearinghouse for processing, and then it is passed along to the patient's health plan provider. If the claim is approved, the health plan provider pays its share for the physician's work, and the necessary adjustments are made based on the explanation of benefits/electronic remittance advice information. Finally, should the remaining balance need to be applied to the patient's coinsurance, a copay, or deductible, the medical biller then bills the patient for any outstanding charges.

**50. C:** Balances that remain unpaid after the first or even second statement is issued are unfortunately common amongst patients and can happen for a variety of reasons. Sending reminder letters and/or additional statements is therefore standard operating procedure for medical billers. If a patient account is nonetheless deemed delinquent after multiple attempts to collect payment, such cases can be turned over to collections agencies. Outstanding patient balances, however, do not accrue interest if they remain unpaid; therefore, if Morgan were to charge interest on the patient's balance, and/or collect such interest on patient payments, she would put herself and the practice at risk for dire consequences during and after an audit. This practice is not only unethical, it is also illegal.

**51. A:** This is a great example of why attention to detail is paramount: Medicare Part B claims can be used for submitting patient claims AND for reporting physician performance data through the Merit-Based Incentive Payment System (MIPS). Additionally, if not written clearly, claim and/or MIPS information can be easily misunderstood when processed by CMS. Modifier 80 is used when surgery is performed with an assistant surgeon; 8P, however, is a MIPS-specific CPT level II modifier used "for [MIPS] reporting purposes only." Issues like the one in the scenario could easily be due to sloppy documentation. The G code tip isn't possible because otologists do not perform audiology services—audiologists do. The suggestion regarding box 24 on the CMS-1500 form is also not possible because it documents the codes for the rendered services being reimbursed and therefore cannot be glossed over. Finally, the UB-04 form, which is like CMS-1500, is used in hospital settings, not in small private practices. A service such as a cochlear implant consultation (versus surgery) could easily be performed in a practice unaffiliated with a hospital, making the use of CMS-1500 appropriate for a Medicare Part B patient claim.

**52. B:** Because this procedure concerns a body part that exists in a pair (i.e., ovaries, oophor-), it is probably a safe assumption that the "×2" can be accounted for through the removal of both (-ectomy). This means that the procedure was not unilateral, but bilateral. Bilateral procedures are most often appended with modifiers to avoid the use of multiple (and unnecessary) codes. Additionally, according to the code-specific guidelines, this procedure can be for EITHER a partial OR a total oophorectomy. If the procedure was truly bilateral, appending "×2" would also make no sense because a woman doesn't have four ovaries. These same guidelines also imply that, unlike many bilateral procedures, this code can be reported without modifiers. This means that it can stand alone, whether bilateral in nature or not. Code 58661 by itself would suffice here for the removal of both ovaries.

**53. D:** This is a coding error that is considered to be double-dipping by the payer; that is, when services already included in one code are separately reported with another code. In this case, when a physician provides the initial casting and subsequent care for a patient's fracture, the two are considered part of the same overall "bundled" service to the patient. This is clearly stipulated in the CPT guidelines for the subsection addressing "Applications of casts and strapping" in the "Musculoskeletal surgery" category.

**54. C:** All independent lab facilities (i.e., those not part of a small physician's office) are required by law to have and to disclose their CLIA numbers, per the federal 1988 Clinical Laboratory Improvement Amendments. Therefore, adding a missing CLIA number is not the correct answer. Modifier 91 is easy to misuse in this field as well—it indicates performing the same lab-based test on the same patient in the same session twice. This modifier is strictly exclusive to exceptional cases and does not apply to scenarios such as confirming the initial results or equipment malfunctions. Codes 81355 and 81535 are services included in the "Pathology and laboratory" section of the CPT, so they can also be removed as possible answers to this question. Modifier QW, however, is a modifier that is ONLY used in small practices, such as physician's offices, where very basic tests requiring no specialized skills can be performed for Medicare patients. An example of a CLIA-waived (i.e., QW) service is an automated dipstick urinalysis.

**55. C:** An ABN, when signed by a Medicare patient, implies that the patient has been informed and understands that a special service or procedure may be denied coverage. This also means that the patient would be financially responsible for covering the cost, if need be, and is agreeing to do so in advance should that be the case. If the service is in fact denied, it's always a good idea to immediately inform the patient as a courtesy before the patient receives the bill.

**56. A:** To start, modifiers LT and RT would never be used in place of modifier 50, so that option is not valid for any carrier. The same logic could be applied to replacing a CPT category I code with a CPT category III code because any and all carriers may be hesitant to cover services and procedures that are experimental and not standardized; therefore, resubmission of a III code in place of an initial I code doesn't make much sense. T codes and G codes, like their LT and RT counterparts, are HCPCS-II codes, which, for the most part, are widely accepted. Some private carriers' guidelines give preference to CPT codes over HCPCS-II codes (unlike Medicare, where HCPCS-II codes are often preferred over the standard CPT, depending on the case). By this logic, resubmission of a T code to a private carrier such as ABC in place of a CPT level I code doesn't seem to be the likely solution; add to this the fact that T codes are specialized to meet the needs of state Medicaid agencies, and all possibility appears gone. However, because Medicare tends to prefer G codes over their CPT equivalents for colorectal screenings, it would make the most sense that ABC probably prefers the opposite. Therefore, resubmitting a CPT I code instead of a G code is the correct answer.

**57. C:** Code 90664 is characterized by an intranasal route of administration, so its use with 90471 is incorrect because 90471 does not account for intranasal administration. In contrast, 90658 is correctly paired with 90471 because both account for intramuscular use; however, the guidelines for vaccines and toxoids in the "Medicine" section of the CPT codebook clearly stipulate that modifier 51 is not to be used with these codes. Code 90680 is correctly paired with 90473, because they both account for an oral route of administration. That said, 90680 is for a rotavirus vaccine, and not an influenza vaccine. Finally, 90660, an influenza code, is correctly paired with codes 90473 and 90474 (an add-on code). This is because 90660 accounts for the vaccine type and 90473 and 90474 account for the corresponding route of administration as well as the number of doses given.

**58. B:** The solution is easily gleaned by looking at the procedure codes included in the "Thyroid excision" coding subsection of the "Endocrine system category" of the CPT codebook. Upon closer scrutiny, there are only two codes listed that include neck dissection: codes 60252 and 60254. The type of neck dissection, limited or radical, is all the coder needs from the doctor. Although there are indeed procedures indicating laterality for thyroid excision, they are clearly not applicable here for coding purposes, nor are any of the isthmusectomy techniques. The use of either code is also not dependent on whether the thyroid removal was total or subtotal because the code descriptors for 60252 and 60254 read "Thyroidectomy, total or subtotal for malignancy."

**59. D:** This question is easily answered by opening up the HCPCS-II codebook and consulting the J codes. Codes J0570 through J0575 pertain to buprenorphine or a mix of buprenorphine with naloxone. Code J0570 is for an implant of 74.2 mg; the implant, however, is for buprenorphine only, not the mixture indicated in the doctor's notes. All medications that *are* mixtures of buprenorphine and naloxone (J0572–J0575) are given orally, so that's not helpful, either. Finally, asking about doses is closer to what the coder needs, but it's not specific enough because the doses are all indicated in milligrams. Therefore, inquiring about the amount of buprenorphine given in milligrams makes the most sense here.

**60. D:** Pain medications will likely produce side effects via somatic and neuronal cells that share the same cell receptors. The side effects, of course, are a direct result of a medication's use of the same biochemical pathway needed for the therapeutic pain relief. So, it would make sense that the doctor would request information about the patient's mental health, medications, allergies, and substance use. Chest x-ray data will probably not help the physician in his decision making. For example, because the physician is already receiving a list of patient allergies (if any), he would already be able to discern whether or not the patient could have adverse allergic reactions to certain medications (e.g., anaphylaxis, which can affect breathing). Consulting chest x-rays would therefore seem redundant.

**61. A:** PHI is generally considered to be any and all patient data that could potentially compromise a patient's identity (and therefore violate their privacy protections under HIPAA). Although a patient's age, DOB, and list of medical conditions are specific to that particular patient, such data alone would not put the patient's identity at risk if it were shared across digital platforms or with the necessary third parties. Disclosure of a patient's full name (or even just a part of it) would be a flagrant violation of HIPAA regulations. Under no reasonable circumstances would the sharing of a patient's full name apply to the minimum necessary data sharing rule. Like sharing a social security number, the disclosure of a name or names within the healthcare system is one of the most dangerous threats to a patient's privacy and security if illicitly exchanged.

**62. C:** The exact definition of a patient-designated record set is always left to a healthcare organization to determine for itself. That said, an overarching theme in healthcare is that patient-designated record sets be directly related to identity-sensitive information protected under HIPAA (claims and billing records, for example). It should be made clear, though, that this general trend does not imply that a covered entity's health record for a patient includes other health records that aren't relevant to the entity's internal administrative purposes and policies. Psychotherapy notes for a patient, for example, would not be included in a record for, say, an orthopedic private practice. Legal notes regarding disputes with patients are also not likely to be found on this record set because the nature of the information may be better suited for the legal health record of the patient. Quality indicator and quality measure reports are not considered HIPAA-sensitive because the data generation for such cases is done in a way that does not compromise the patient's PHI. Patient claims and billing records, however, would be a treasure trove of PHI to access for anyone with ill intentions. Covered entities are thus generally known to include such (HIPAA-protected) data in designated record sets for patients.

**63. C:** When it comes to HIPAA-protected information, the basic building blocks of data considered to be inherently sensitive to patient privacy and security regulations (a social security number, for example) are made even more sensitive through the context in which they are documented. This is why the information (PHI) contained on a medical claim or record, for example, would be desirable for hackers and identity thieves. The more PHI that is documented in one place, the more dangerous it is to expose to eyes not meant to see it. There are overlaps, though. A patient's full name could either be sensitive PHI or much less sensitive patient-identifiable information, depending on the context in which it is it being used. So, the statement regarding the two as being the same is inherently false. PHI cannot legally be disclosed to just anyone, but patient-identifiable data could be disclosed in some contexts; therefore, it would make more sense to encrypt PHI if it is, in fact, shared (and not the other way around). The statement regarding the OIG is also false; the use of patient-identifiable data for administrative purposes is not necessarily exclusive. Anyone working an administrative role in a doctor's office could potentially see such data. Therefore, although there may be overlap between some basic data that could fall under either PHI or administrative, patient-identifiable data, the risk to patient privacy depends entirely on the context through which they are used and/or shared.

**64. A:** Quantitative deficiencies in patient records have less to do with actual numeric data and more to do with record completeness—crucial data that are either incomplete or missing. If all required data fields needed are full (i.e., they are complete, even if incorrect), then any numeric errors, errors of a careless nature, and even overall patient data quantity would fall into the qualitative data category. A quantitative deficiency could easily be identified if a patient's DOB is missing a year or if it includes a year but contains two digits instead of four. Another quantitative deficiency could be identified if a medicated patient's new insurance plan data are mostly intact, but his or her new Rx BIN number field was not recorded. It is important to note that even if the Rx BIN number is visible in the scanned image of the new insurance card, its empty corresponding field in the patient database would still be a deficiency. An image alone cannot be readily searched or mined for patient data but a corresponding alphanumeric-based index of patient data can be.

**65. C:** Varicella (chickenpox), MMR, and meningitis vaccines are generally administered to Americans while they are still young. Doing so helps the US population maintain its herd immunity and therefore prevent any public health emergencies related to outbreaks. Different populations of people throughout the world tend to also share immunity (and susceptibility) to certain diseases. They do, of course, vary between populations, and so any individual (such as an international student) who enters into a population other than his or her own (such as the US) is at risk for contracting certain diseases and for spreading them. Therefore, requiring students to have the necessary vaccinations (such as those mentioned above) shields the student's health and the health of other students. Not having an HPV vaccination, however, would not pose a significant threat to either the student or the people that he or she comes into contact with. It is extremely rare for HPV to be life-threatening (causing cervical cancer, for example), and it is not known to cause outbreaks, even though it is viral and has many different types. Thus, in this particular context, lacking proof of an HPV vaccination would not be considered a quantitative deficiency on an international student vaccination record.

**66. C:** The deficiency of concern in this section of the report has to do with Kristin's insurance information. Although she is on file as a Consolidated Omnibus Budget Reconciliation Act (COBRA) beneficiary, it would be appropriate for the billing department to give her a call and determine her insurance status. This is because the use of COBRA benefits is only valid for six months. Because Kristin was laid off in mid-January of the same year that this report was generated, her intermediary coverage has technically been expired now for a week. Giving her a call and adding a note to her file would probably be a good idea, depending on where she is in the job search process.

**67. D:** Xanax is a commonly prescribed benzodiazepine for persons who are prone to severe anxiety and panic attacks. Because of their powerful (and often immediate) therapeutic effects on the autonomic nervous system, this class of drug is highly addictive and extremely dangerous in high doses. A 15 mg dose per day, or even as needed, is unheard of and is incredibly dangerous to patient safety. What probably happened here was that the person documenting the prescription list forgot to use a decimal point—1.5 mg falls within the recommended 0.5–2.0 mg range for daily use. Additionally, such an error in documentation would be considered to be qualitative (versus quantitative) because the numeric digits used are correct, but the manner in which they were initially recorded is not.

**68. C:** A discharge status (e.g., alive, deceased), although certainly applicable, would probably be least useful to the survey because it is already implied that the data being collected are all coming from those deceased due to COVID-19. Because it was still a relatively new disease in the United States in 2020, any and all information that could lead to patterns and trends of the disease's etiology and manifestation would be most useful. This included such data fields as admission or referral source, patient ethnicity and race, sex, knowledge of any known underlying medical conditions, time and date of onset to time and date of death, and age at death, among many others.

**69. D:** For refugees coming to the United States from a third-world country, known (or suspected) cases of diseases such as rickets (a severe vitamin D deficiency common in malnourished populations) or malaria (a parasitic disease caused by mosquitoes) are known to be life-threatening and would require immediate medical attention. Women who are pregnant would also necessitate an in-depth evaluation: depending on the mother's health, a delivery could also potentially be life-threatening, and care would need to be taken to ensure the survival of the mother and child. By contrast, myopia is an eye condition that we know colloquially as nearsightedness. Because it is not a life-threatening disease or condition, it would most likely not be prioritized among the list of the refugees' most immediate healthcare needs.

**70. C:** The dietitian and psychotherapist can easily be eliminated from possible resources to the counselor because neither one is considered to be a practicing physician. Primary care providers, who are physicians, certainly keep lists of their patients' medications on hand for consultation, but they generally don't prescribe medication unless the patient has a transient condition (such as an infection) that can be treated with a temporary remedy (e.g., an antibiotic). Additionally, because the supplement clearly involves the production of neurotransmitters, this is an area of expertise that the primary care physician is probably not qualified to address or treat. A psychiatrist, however, is, so this would be the best go-to person for the counselor.

**71. B:** Preoperative x-rays, cancer treatment records, and a list of current medications are all relevant to the orthopedic surgeon's understanding of the patient's needs. Anesthetic allergies are also relevant, but there's a problem: the anesthetics involved in monitored anesthesia care (MAC) are not applicable to hip replacement surgery. Such a surgery would actually require general anesthesia (i.e., the patient is completely unconscious), not MAC services (i.e., the patient is only sedated and locally anesthetized while completely conscious). Although it is true that anesthetic allergies must be taken into account ahead of time, a much simpler route to this information would be to request a list of known allergies, which should include anesthetic allergies. Requesting allergy information for an anesthesiology procedure that isn't applicable to the surgery in question would be of little (if any) use to the surgeon. A simple list of all known allergies would also better serve the minimum necessary standard for requesting new-patient PHI from third-party healthcare entities.

**72. C:** An EMPI, which can also be understood as an overarching umbrella PI for all master patient indexes (MPIs) within a healthcare system, is used for maintaining the accuracy, completeness, and integrity of patient records for a multitude of purposes. It contains every piece of patient data related to the patient's own unique history of healthcare treatment, planning, and outcomes. It is a well-known fact that all such patient records need to be kept within an MPI or EMPI for at least 10 years, if not indefinitely, unless state regulations stipulate otherwise. Records of patient visits to different covered entity types within a system (i.e., clinics, hospitals, outpatient centers, etc., or "verticals") would therefore be expected. Because these verticals all contain their own patient identifiers in addition to a master patient ID used for cross-referencing, duplicates are common; therefore, flagging software is a necessary component of a well-maintained system. Finally, although patient data can certainly be used for compliance and auditing purposes, compliance and auditing data have no place in an MPI. This is because data mining for such purposes may only indirectly (as opposed to directly) influence future patient care, thereby potentially impacting the nature and scope of future data entries.

**73. B:** Part of the 1996 HIPAA legislation instituted what is known as a national patient identification system, which assigned one unique record identifier for every American receiving healthcare. The identifier, once issued, is permanent, in life and in death (mostly for legal purposes). This federal regulation was meant to help create a more uniform, streamlined patient health record because the use of multiple patient identifiers had left most records fragmented and only accessible in chunks. In actual practice today, of course, it's still not a foolproof system, but most healthcare administrators can agree that it was a step in the right direction.

**74. C:** In the outpatient setting, J codes, or those codes specific to drugs, biologicals and, in some cases, chemotherapeutic agents, are not reported if the facility itself did not purchase the drug. Conversely, in those instances in which the drug or substance being administered was purchased by the facility, then it is reported. However, only the facility can bill for the administration of the drug, never the provider. This means that practicing physicians in this setting should never be encouraged to report the drugs they give, which also applies to an emergency department, for example. Although located at a hospital, it is not considered an inpatient setting and therefore is an outpatient setting by default. Drug application and dosage are also imperative details that cannot be overlooked in coding/reporting because both pieces of information are needed for Medicare to confirm (or deny) the medical necessity of the service being rendered on a claim.

**75. D:** Reporting the appropriate codes for vaccination encounters is dependent on the route of administration because a J code might be on a drug's mode of application. Unlike J codes, however, vaccine codes all require a minimum of two total codes: one for the vaccine type itself and another for the route in which it is given (intramuscular versus subcutaneous, for example). Any vaccine codes that follow the initial two are always either add-on codes for the vaccine given or are completely different codes documenting the administration of another vaccine that was given within the same session. For such patient encounters, it is also common knowledge that vaccinations are totally age-dependent due to their direct correlation with blood serum toxicity risks (among many other potential complications). This is why a person's age will always affect the type of vaccine given, as well as the dosage. Counseling, although often given, is not always given; as a result, some vaccine codes have two variations: one that includes counseling and another that does not (care should be taken to differentiate between them). Although counseling could have always been given separately during a previously scheduled encounter, counseling followed by a shot within the same session is quite common. The following should be noted, however: if the only reason for a visit is to get vaccinated, no E/M code is reported—doing so constitutes "unbundling" services that are not meant to be reported separately.

**76. A:** The case mix index is a standard measure for CMS when determining and/or recalibrating reimbursement rates in hospitals and/or other facilities. Although certain healthcare variables such as patient mortality, durations of patient stays, and coding workflow/accuracy are not unimportant, a case mix index analysis considers many fluctuating individual variables related to patient care when a situation calls for new measures. Once these are all entered into a fixed algorithm, CMS can then determine the appropriate measures needed to holistically address ongoing changes and trends in patient care.

**77. C:** Data regarding patient treatment histories, as well as the place of treatment (inpatient or outpatient), certainly matter to a cancer drug study, but these data are more likely to be collected before the first phase of the trial begins in order to select and target the population most in need of the drug, albeit experimentally. It would make more sense to gather data on adverse reactions and side effects across the initial population studied as the appropriate dosages and toxicity thresholds are determined, and possibly even adjusted. It would therefore make no sense to administer placebos.

**78. A:** The laceration of popliteal artery code is correct, but the diagnostic context of this code is incomplete. Per the coding note found under category S85.0, "S" must be appended at the end of the code to indicate the context of the patient's visit as well as the nature of the documented injury (i.e., "sequela"). This results in a code that should read S85.019S. (The "S" preceding the code only indicates that the diagnosis code comes from Chapter 19 of the ICD-10.)

**79. D:** Code 88346 seems to be the correct code, but there are a few problems. First of all, performing a staining service on multiple specimens is standard for CLIA-certified laboratories. Therefore, the use of modifier 22, "increased procedural services," is inappropriate because such procedures are generally just used with their respective add-on codes. Code 88350 is the corresponding add-on code for 88346; but when indicated with an "×3," the overall code set would imply staining four specimens, versus the three indicated. Additionally, there is a parenthetical note below add-on code 88350 that reads "Do not report 88346 and 88350 for fluorescent in situ hybridization studies," and then it lists more appropriate codes. Among such codes is 88365, fluorescent in situ hybridization. Its corresponding add-on code is 88364; however, the use of add-on codes with modifier 51 not permitted. Plus, the added implication of "multiple procedures," such as "increased procedural services," does not make sense in this context. Therefore, the correct code set is 88365, 88364×2.

**80. C:** The easiest and most efficient way to answer this question is to turn to Appendix E in the back of the CPT codebook, the "Summary of CPT Codes Exempt from Modifier 51." According to the index description, "This ... list of [procedure codes] are typically exempt from multiple procedure reductions." Codes 20697, 61107, and 93612 are all on that list; code 11200 is not.

**81. C:** As a basic rule of thumb, place-of-service codes that are incorrectly assigned on medical claims are generally returned to the sender for correction. In large hospitals in which coders/billers are often expected to generate high volumes of claims, it is easy—especially when under stress—to make mistakes. At the front of the CPT codebook is a list of place-of-service codes that are organized numerically from 01 to 99. Upon consultation of this list, the place-of-service codes 02, 25, and 23 are assigned appropriately; code 12, however, corresponds to "Home," which is clearly incorrect, due to the nature of the services reported (i.e., performed in an intensive care unit). The correct code is 21, "Inpatient hospital." Judging by the fact that both codes use the same two numbers, the person generating the claim probably had the right code in mind, but just entered the two digits in the wrong order. This is a mistake that could be easily made if he or she was in a hurry or had a strict quota deadline to meet, for example. If someone is available to check claims for accuracy, it could make a great difference in the workload volume and efficiency of the billing department because new claims are always being made and any that aren't properly documented are sent back for correction.

**82. D:** Although the encounter is for a simple routine wellness check, the place of service (a temporary group living home) takes precedence over the type of service (preventative medicine). Therefore, applying preventative medicine service 99387 would be incorrect. Modifier 96, "Habilitative services," is also inappropriate, because it doesn't apply to a (physical) wellness check, and the fact that the (albeit disabled) patient lives in a group home would be self-evident in the use of the appropriate E/M code in "Home services." A letter would also not be appropriate here because the coder must strictly adhere to the data received. As such, the coder would need to explain to the physician that although the encounter was highly stressful and took far longer than normal, 99345 would still not apply from a time standpoint, nor would the "high complexity" of the medical decision making involved—especially because there were no abnormal findings. The coder would also have to clarify that 99345 requires a "comprehensive" history and exam, which clearly don't apply to a basic physical evaluation. However difficult the execution of these services may have been due to the patient's preexisting behavioral issues, such issues nonetheless do not apply to the coding criteria for this E/M category. Therefore, because Medicare clearly wouldn't cover the services rendered for 99345, the coder would probably recommend that 99341 be reported instead.

**83. B:** Whatever the supervising physician's reasons were for reporting physician-only codes for a nonphysician (perhaps in this case bending the rules out of guilt for the unusual extenuating circumstances) a coder's allegiance is first and foremost to the known data for a patient encounter. Therefore, if it is known that a resident performed services without the direct supervision of a physician, physician-only codes cannot and will not apply. A letter would be a waste of time because CMS would reject the claim with or without one. Reporting the codes on two separate occasions is also illegal and makes the coder just as liable for enabling fraudulent behavior as the doctor. Reporting the doctor's actions to his own board is also completely unnecessary (and inappropriate because it is outside the scope of a coder's responsibilities). All the coder has to do is explain to the physician that the codes reported would be considered fraudulent, no matter the circumstances of the encounter. Although the situation was indeed unfortunate for the resident, the coder must maintain his or her position as the "gatekeeper" of data integrity between physicians (including physicians-to-be) and CMS.

**84. B:** In documentation, the type of diabetes is always useful, but it is not required—the default for a coder is E11 (type 2). (Ideally, the more specific, the better, but this doesn't always happen.) In the ICD-10 index, look for "Neuropathy." In this category there is a subcategory that says "Peripheral," and then another, "Autonomic," and finally, "Diabetes mellitus – see E08-E13 with .43." Many potential diagnoses are found with slight variations—two being E08.43, "Diabetes mellitus due to underlying condition with diabetic autonomic neuropathy," and E09.43, "Drug- or chemical-induced diabetes mellitus with … autonomic polyneuropathy." The diabetes flowchart in the ICD-10 guidelines equally indicates that the type and cause of the diabetes are crucial to the final code assignment. A patient's blood glucose reading (A1C), although common for monitoring purposes in diabetic patients, is not a criterion considered by a payer when determining medical necessity in such cases; therefore, it is of no real use in assigning diagnosis codes.

**85. A:** For this procedure to be documented correctly, code 70540 is reported alone because it does not need any modifiers, and it should only be reported once. It is true that for this particular code type, modifiers 26 and TC could potentially represent the two parts of one whole procedure: TC is for the use of the necessary equipment (the technical component), and 26 is the postprocedural interpretation of results (the professional component). Indeed, if two professionals perform each part of the procedure separately, then reporting the code twice with its associated modifiers (70540-26, 70540-TC) would be appropriate. However, the tech did not participate in the procedure, and her presence is not enough to warrant credit for the work that is due solely to the doctor. That said, reporting 70540-TC-26 for the physician's work is equally erroneous because it is inherently redundant. Finally, because it is not uncommon for in-house hospital radiologists to perform both procedural components when necessary, such services would not constitute billable extra time and effort, making 70540-22 incorrect.

**86. B:** Most coders' go-to resource for coding-related updates, changes, and releases is CMS (cms.gov). However, if one is interested in CPT-only updates, the AMA (ama-assn.org) is the best resource. This is because the AMA is responsible for CPT coding updates and changes. The FDA (fda.gov), although responsible for approving CPT, is not considered a primary resource for CPT coding changes. The resources available from the CDC (cdc.gov), such as a comprehensive disease index, would probably be a better supplementary resource to the ICD-10-CM. Finally, the OIG (oig.hhs.gov) is completely unrelated to coding regulations. It would better serve as a reference point for human resources-related needs; compliance planning; and external auditing information for hospitals, clinics, and private practices.

**87. C:** CPT Appendix B lists all up-to-date code changes made from the previous year only. With regard to the latest annual category I coding updates, the AMA or CMS are easily accessible resources. Levels II and III code change information may also be found there, although they do not run on the same update schedule as their category I counterparts. The most easily accessible guide to these individual update schedules (running anywhere from biannually to quarterly) can be found in the back foldout of the CPT manual.

**88. D:** As a basic rule of thumb, coding guidelines are always the primary resource for any inquiries regarding sequencing rules. This would be especially true for any new codes or code categories (such as those related to COVID-19). Supplementary tables for the tabular list and index are useful for penciling in new materials within the ICD-10, but they would only really assist a coder with where to find these new codes. A conversion table, by contrast, is far more extensive and includes code adjustments for all viral and microbial-related diseases—not just COVID-19. Coding descriptions in tabular order could be useful for sequencing, but only if there are any applicable notes (such as "Use additional code," "Code also," etc.). These notes, however, would still only be secondary to any and all newly released guidelines that address all sequencing rules directly.

**89. D:** Codes Z11.52, Z86.16, and D84.9 are the most appropriate codes, and they are also sequenced correctly. Even when armed with only an ICD-10 codebook that doesn't yet contain the new codes, one could still determine that these are the best codes through the application of basic logic. This is accomplished primarily through a coder's own familiarity with code categories (organized by letter) and by consulting the old codes given within their subclassifications (which also correspond to the new codes). To start, because the patient is presenting for a screening, an experienced coder knows that it will be a Z code. There are three given in the new code set. If one begins with the old code Z11.59, we see that it is listed under "Z11 – Encounter for screening for infectious and parasitic diseases," and then it is subcategorized further under "Z11.5 – Encounter for screening for other viral diseases." Therefore, code Z11.52 applies; however, the reasons for the encounter make the remaining code selections more difficult to navigate. Because Z20.822 would be listed similarly to the old code Z20.828, in which both would be categorized under "Z20.8 – Contact with and (suspected) exposure to other communicable diseases," it can be eliminated as a potential code because it is known that the patient has a congenital immunosuppressive condition, D84.9, a fact that should also be present in the code report submitted due to the possibility that it will affect the test administration. Then, when further comparing J12.82 to Z86.16, the final answer becomes most evident: J is clearly an illness code ("J12 – Viral pneumonia, not elsewhere classified") versus Z86.16, which is a history code ("Z86.1 – Personal history of infectious and parasitic diseases"). Because it is known that the patient contracted COVID-19 in the past (pneumonic or not), it is the most logical choice here to justify the medical necessity of the encounter alongside code D84.9.

**90. C:** R91.8 is correct because it is indicated that the physician *suspects* pulmonary eosinophilia, but that doesn't mean he knows for sure that this is the case. He is likely running several tests before a more specific diagnosis is certain. He therefore documents the condition for the time being as "pulmonary infiltrate NOS." Additionally, if one consults the tabular list for "pulmonary eosinophilia," the coder is led to J82—one of the conditions listed by the CDC as related to, or resulting from, vaping activity. That said, if J82 is examined more closely, there is a note at the very bottom of EXCLUDES 1 that reads: "pulmonary infiltrate NOS (R91.8)." This means that the patient may very well have the condition suspected, but because it is not known yet, this is the closest diagnosis code to what is already known for sure. Finally, R07.9 and R06.00 are the symptoms that the patient presented with; however, when a diagnosis (however vague) is documented, symptoms are not. These R codes would have been appropriate codes had the patient presented with these symptoms and the admitting physician had not yet determined a diagnosis.

**91. B:** $49.19 is the correct answer.

$$\begin{aligned}
\text{FPA} &= [(0.95 \times 1.000) + (0.39 \times 0.992) + (0.06 \times 1.088)] \times \$35.0785 \\
&= [(0.95) + (0.38688) + (0.06528)] \times \$35.0785 \\
&= [1.40216] \times \$35.0785 \\
&= \$49.19
\end{aligned}$$

$69.79 is incorrect—this results when 0.6 is factored into the formula instead of the given 0.06.
$48.23 is incorrect—this results when 0.922 is factored into the formula instead of the given 0.992.
$50.85 is incorrect—this results when 1.88 is factored into the formula instead of the given 1.088.

**92. A:** $107.39 is the correct answer.

$$\begin{aligned}
\text{NFPA} &= [0.92 \times 1.5 + 1.85 \times 1.029 + 0.07 \times 0.0791] \times \$32.1618 \\
&= [1.38 + 1.90365 + 0.05537] \times \$32.1618 \\
&= 3.33902 \times \$32.1618 \\
&= \$107.39
\end{aligned}$$

$123.42 is incorrect—this results when 0.7 is factored into the formula instead of the given 0.07.
$118.10 is incorrect—this results when 1.209 is factored into the formula instead of the given 1.029.
$107.79 is incorrect—this results when 0.971 is factored into the formula instead of the given 0.791.

**93. A:** As a general rule when assigning E/M codes, physicians are always encouraged to select the HIPAA guidelines that: 1) offer the best framework for justifying medical necessity and any associated note taking, 2) best characterize the nature of the encounter, and 3) best remunerate the doctor within the confines of the first two criteria. That said, anything that well documents the medical necessity of an encounter alone tends to be the best way to justify code selection. The second statement about "gray areas" is false because it is, in fact, on the contrary: it is well known that the very reason for the 1997 guideline release was because the 1995 guidelines were criticized as being too vague. The third statement is also switched: because the 1997 guidelines offer much more specific parameters for documenting an exam, they are actually much better suited to note taking—especially because it encourages the use of bulleted data (an organizational feature that the 1995 guidelines do not contain). Documentation—its structure, organization, and content—is often what makes or breaks coverage approval; so much so that different carriers may require data that fit within the construct of their own definitions. This makes the last statement totally false—carriers tend NOT to agree on what constitutes "limited," "extended," or "complete" exams. It is therefore imperative that the guidelines of each patient's carrier are taken into consideration before E/M codes and their corresponding documentation are submitted.

**94. A:** CPT infusion codes are easy to miscode because most service and/or procedure codes are reported per day of service within a single patient encounter. Infusion codes are an exception to this rule, especially because it is common for them to overlap between calendar days. There is a good example given to demonstrate the proper use of these codes in the CPT section "Medicine." The hydration infusion guidelines read as follows: "[i]f intravenous hydration (96360, 96361) is given from 11 PM to 2 AM, 96360 would be reported once [initial infusion of 31–60 minutes] and 96361 twice [each hour following initial administration]." Reporting the wrong type of infusion (chemotherapy versus hydration, for example) is certainly possible but not all that likely. The use of modifiers regarding administrating staff versus doctors is not an existing coding standard and is therefore false; the guidelines themselves further stipulate that such codes are "not intended to be reported by the physician or other qualified healthcare professional in the facility setting." Finally, the 31-minute rule used for prepping a patient for chemotherapy is a known standard operating procedure in which hydration time cannot be compromised (i.e., fewer than 31 minutes). This is mostly due to the potential (including legal) ramifications for the facility if a cancer patient is inappropriately medicated. Therefore, miscoding is not at all likely if the required duration is clearly documented.

**95. C:** Compliance officers within a healthcare practice are tasked primarily with providing the leadership necessary to ensure ethical and efficient compliance plan development, execution, and review. Even if the workplace is not expecting an external audit from the OIG, the best compliance officers will implement a clear, policy-based infrastructure that is completely integrated into the standard operating procedures of the workplace. By doing so, the established compliance procedures and standards become second nature to all involved and the potential stress generated within that workplace is minimized when audits are performed. The compliance officer is equipped with many OIG-based resources that guide his or her compliance planning and management in preparation for a potential audit; however, the OIG does not require participation in its national project development initiatives.

**96. D:** Corrective action for compliance violations will vary depending on the healthcare practice and the compliance policies that it has implemented to ensure best practices. Enforcing violation procedures is always a given when noncompliance is discovered; such corrective actions can range from issuing a refund to reporting criminal activity. A lawsuit is a potential course of action in the most extreme cases; however, the compliance officer would probably not be given exclusive access to OIG lawyers. It would be far more efficient (and appropriate) for the officer to call the OIG and request a referral for a lawyer within his or her particular locale.

**97. B:** Semantic data acquire significant value beyond their own base definition due to the context in which they are framed and presented on the EHR. This means that semantic data can, in fact, include and encompass many, if not all, categories of patient data (qualitative, quantitative, previously validated, etc.). The individual values of such data will, of course, naturally vary from patient to patient, although all data should be archived within a standardized health record framework and structure that encompasses the entirety of the patient's healthcare history. The resulting body of original information is thus easier to maintain and interpret for the purposes of maximizing the quality of patient care, as well as the integrity of the information and the institution responsible for storing it.

**98. C:** It is important to differentiate between encoders and coders. Encoders are digital coding tools. Encoders may or may not be used by coders, who are people charged with responsibly and accurately translating patient report data into predetermined alphanumeric codes. This is done in order to best facilitate billing and reimbursement services. Encoders are becoming an integral tool for coders in healthcare—at least for those who have access to them. Computer-assisted coding (CAC) software programs, for example, contain built-in encoders as critical central components to their overall operation by the coders using them. In theory, they are meant to increase output by decreasing the time spent on each patient report while maintaining a high rate of coding accuracy.

**99. D:** A practice management system is a software program or platform that helps regulate the business of healthcare rather than the healthcare itself. The hands-on side of healthcare—spearheaded primarily by physicians, rather than facility administrators—is nowadays best assisted through the use of an EHR. When researching EHR system programs, an interface that makes report writing easy and whose overall infrastructure maximizes patient care quality is important to consider. An EHR would not be integrated into a practice management system, however. Doing so would likely disrupt the facility workflow due to inefficiently structured information silos shared between those who manage the logistics of healthcare versus those actually providing it. Therefore, when researching the practice management systems available on the market, simple administrative tools such as a calendar/scheduler would be more pertinent to the needs of the IT and HIM sphere of the healthcare workforce.

**100. B:** The reason that a software's output is only as good as its input is because of the garbage in, garbage out principle. This means that the software's coding quality is only ever as good as the quality of the data that it is given. This is especially true of a doctor, say, who doesn't take good notes on his patient reports —or at least doesn't give the bot the input it needs to algorithmically derive the best codes necessary for the encounter. If this is done over time, it compounds the integrity of the software's output. Even worse, if the patient's medical record is missing information, is incongruous in any way, or is organized into fields incompatible with the bot's analytic features, the probability of potential software errors also compounds quickly and easily if not rectified properly. Consequently, the healthcare world will always need coders, regardless of the prevalence of CAC software. A coder can not only directly influence (and improve) the bot's artificial intelligence data memory bank with corrections, but can also indirectly improve its output integrity by flagging flaws in the patient record for the HIM department's rectification. Although it is certainly not perfect in practice, in theory, such a workflow model could drastically improve digital patient data quality and streamlining for CAC-based coding needs.

**101. B:** As a general rule in coding, simplifying is always preferable if the situation allows for it. This is especially true of combination codes. Although the physician indeed documented the patient's symptoms as separate from one another, it is actually best practice (and also far more efficient) to use combination codes when available for symptoms often occurring together, rather than to list them all individually. In this case, nausea should be coded with vomiting using the available combination code R11.2. Likewise, fever with chills should also be coded using combination code R50.9. Doing so would teach the autocoder in the CAC software how to handle such documentation in the future. Additionally, the coder could educate the physician about how to best electronically document common (and sometimes co-occurring) symptoms to increase workflow efficiency. For example, documenting the same set of symptoms as "1. Fever with chills and 2. Nausea with vomiting" would have probably made it easier for the CAC to recognize data corresponding to combination codes instead of individual codes.

**102. A:** Giving a physician written permission to share PHI with a third party is only fully authorized by law when the patient fills out a HIPAA release form. A patient giving written permission to do so by any other means (including an email) is just as unlawful as giving a physician oral permission out loud during a session together. Patients who are at least 18 years old are protected by law through HIPAA; therefore, the only way to waive this right is to do so through HIPAA itself. The other three scenarios represent the proper handling of patient PHI under HIPAA regulations. Nondisclosure of a patient's whereabouts (such as a psychiatric facility) is standard best practice as is complying with a patient's preferences with regard to how he or she wishes to have PHI disclosed. A primary care physician requesting a new patient's medical history can also be justified through the "medical necessity" rule: it helps guide the new doctor's treatment of that patient within the parameters of his or her own healthcare history, therefore maximizing the quality and effectiveness of the patient's (new) ongoing care.

**103. C:** Unless the patient gives express permission in writing, under no circumstances can a healthcare provider share any part of a patient's health record, period. This is what HIPAA protects against: the sharing of patient information that could potentially compromise his or her safety and security if accessed illicitly. It is the job of the healthcare provider to maintain integrity as a practitioner by refraining from such action; whether the patient is honest or dishonest about their vaccine status in the public or private sphere is not of concern. That said, if a patient gets in legal trouble due to PHI fraud (such as falsifying their own vaccination record), educating providers on what happens legally during such scenarios would probably be very useful and could even assist in developing patient education materials on the subject. The "are you vaccinated?" question could also be discussed in such materials—it is not illegal to inquire of someone face-to-face about their vaccination status because it doesn't involve the illicit sharing of electronic PHI. (Besides, the patient has the right to answer or refuse to answer per their HIPAA rights.) Finally, regarding vaccine passports, it is inherently assumed that whoever has such a passport is using it to voluntarily disclose their vaccine status in order to travel. As long as a patient is sharing his or her own vaccination status for such means, HIPAA is a nonissue.

**104. B:** Adding foreign language on top of patient HIPAA rights can easily complicate any scenario in a healthcare setting. In this case, as long as the patient's PHI is not exclusively shared with anyone other than the patient, violations are highly unlikely. An educational pamphlet is not problematic because the patient still has the power to choose to share it or keep it private. Rescheduling an appointment with a phone interpreter or having someone assist the patient with understanding the reason she can't be seen also do not compromise a patient's PHI. However, calling home for an interpreting request is inappropriate on several counts. First of all, it is disclosed that the patient never signed any HIPAA release forms at the clinic, which inherently implies that, by law, her PHI cannot be shared with anyone. Simply identifying the patient's current whereabouts over the phone is a privacy breach. Secondly, using a family member to translate results for the patient implies that PHI will be shared with someone other than just the patient. Thirdly, it presents a potential conflict of interest that would put the patient's healthcare at risk for misunderstanding or misinformation—an issue easily avoided with a professional interpreter with no personal involvement with the patient.

**105. C:** Using a thumb drive for personal files on a work-only computer containing patient-sensitive data would likely not be in the agreement due to the HIPAA security risks involved in doing so. This is because it would be easy for the medical assistant to use the USB key to copy and paste patient data from the hard drive to the thumb drive without a trace of wrongdoing. (Fact: laptop hard drive encryption software keeps data encrypted ONLY when they stay in the hard drive; the encryption would not extend to other storage mediums if copied or transferred outside of it.) Including a clause in the security agreement stipulating that legal action would be taken for information transferred to other media without the proper authorization may also not deter someone from wrongdoing. Therefore, although it seems like a smart idea on the surface, in most cases, any healthcare HR manager would see such "personal" use of external information technology as too risky.

**106. B:** It is common (and best) practice to have passwords that are randomly generated and therefore cannot easily be memorized. This is usually accomplished with the use of a combination of characters across different categories. That said, other than the use of the infamous "password," the use of numeric sequences such as "12345" is another obvious (and easily avoided) security vulnerability. Although numbers are certainly recommended for use in passwords along with special characters and upper- and lowercase letters, it is best that they be randomly placed and selected rather than put in a sequence that anyone can remember.

**107. D:** The minimum necessary standard applies to protecting sensitive patient data (PHI). This means that the name and address of a physician, or even a lab CLIA number, likely poses little, if any, security risk to the patient specimens in question. Complete results of a pathology report are certainly sensitive; however, it is a "necessary" piece of data in this instance because the use of the document is for scientifically based research. A patient's ID number—especially if it is transferred to the lab from the hospital when the referral is initially made—is definitely sensitive. Depending on the nature of the electronic trail that it reveals, it could be the key that opens the door to additional pieces of PHI. It is therefore best that it be blacked out or encrypted when the reports are shared.

**108. B:** The HIM Department is where all patient release forms should be submitted once signed. An HIM professional knows best how to authorize, process, store, and protect the integrity of the information to be shared. The other three acronyms are easy to eliminate because they are not departments at all. HIT stands for health information technology—a necessary HIM tool. The EHR is the patient's electronic health record (versus his or her paper record). Finally, IGPHC stands for Information Governance Principles for Healthcare—a national standard for patient data archiving that all healthcare entities are expected to honor and uphold. This is done through the development of internal policies governing the quality, organization, storage, and security of patient and administrative records.

**109. A:** PHI is required by law (HIPAA) to be stored and shared securely between digital interfaces, and most of the time this is done through encryption. Although employment/insurance history, sociodemographic information, age and sex data may not implicitly be considered as PHI on their own, such data could nonetheless cross over into PHI territory if the context in which they are documented creates a potential vulnerability to the patient's identity and/or privacy.

**110. D:** Cloud storage technology has become hugely popular due to its ability to limit data storage on computer hard drives, resulting in smoother machine operation and better overall performance health. Unfortunately, because this technology is still a relatively new one, it isn't foolproof. Cloud services generally include encryption in their software or platform programs, but a cloud's overall security, encrypted or not, is only as good as the robustness of its accessibility pathways. Therefore, any cloud technology that allows for a person to share data directly in an unsecured link implies that it is not as secure as it may market itself to be.

**111. B:** Leaving patient PHI on a Post-it Note would be a HIPAA violation in most (if not all) circumstances. Such open (and dangerous) exposure of sensitive patient data certainly does not fit the privacy/security protection requirements stipulated by HIPAA. It would also violate the minimum necessary standard: PHI, when shared (securely as opposed to openly), is only ever meant for those few people responsible for making the healthcare transactions needed in medically necessary circumstances regarding a patient's care. Although the person with the Post-it Note at the computer may be one of those people, chances are that the people working in and around that person's workspace are not.

**112. B:** Although it is true that most patient information in healthcare has gone mostly digital, retaining paper records is still not uncommon. Should that be the case, hiring a company that specializes in secure shredding is the best way to destroy confidential documents. Normally, this involves obtaining a specialized dumpster that medical records cannot be taken back out of once they are placed in it. The company owning the dumpster then takes care of the shredding and destruction of the documents. Shredding and trashing in house, although mostly secure, still runs the risk of information being stolen—either by people who shouldn't be doing the shredding or by others looking to steal information from the trash.

# CCA Practice Test #2

**1. Which of the following is NOT an acceptable method for destroying confidential medical records?**
   a. Placing them in a medical waste container
   b. Shredding, pulverizing, incinerating, and pulping
   c. Digital sanitation
   d. Transferring them to a disposal vendor

**2. A patient is seen first by the medical assistant, who documents a body mass index (BMI) of 36, a history of nicotine dependence, and a blood pressure reading of 140/85. The physician later documents a diagnosis of hypertension. What code(s) should be reported for this encounter?**
   a. I10
   b. I10, Z87.891
   c. I10, E66.9, Z68.36, Z87.891
   d. I10, Z68.36, Z87.891

**3. Which of the following actions is a violation of the AHIMA Standards of Ethical Coding?**
   a. A query was sent to a physician to confirm a diagnosis of suspected *Escherichia coli* urinary tract infection.
   b. A patient was seen for birth control and pelvic pain. Birth control is not covered under the patient's insurance; therefore, only pelvic pain is reported on the claim.
   c. An online search engine was used to locate a diagnosis code for thickened endometrium.
   d. Unsolicited advice was provided to educate physicians on correct documentation.

**4. Which diagnosis requires that additional data be abstracted from the health record?**
   a. Chronic kidney disease
   b. Postprocedural hypothyroidism
   c. Acute schizophrenia
   d. Tinea corporis

**5. A primary care physician may request records from a patient's endocrinologist without obtaining a patient's authorization under which of the following laws?**
   a. Online Privacy Protection Act
   b. HIPAA Privacy Rule
   c. Privacy Act of 1974
   d. Gramm-Leach-Bliley Act

**6. "Patient is seen with complaints of melena and dark, tarry stool. Suspect possible upper GI hemorrhage. Patient sent to ED for further evaluation." What diagnosis code(s) should be reported?**
   a. K92.1, R19.5
   b. K92.2
   c. K92.2, K92.1, R19.5
   d. K92.1

7. A large bowel partial resection was performed on a patient through an abdominal incision. What CPT code should be reported?
   a. 44140
   b. 45379
   c. 44204
   d. 44210

8. A physician performs a right shoulder surgical arthroscopy to repair a chronic torn rotator cuff. During the procedure, the physician determines that he needs more room to work and converts to an open procedure. How should the physician report the procedure(s)?
   a. 23412
   b. 23412, 29827-51
   c. 23410
   d. 23410, 29827-51

9. Which of the following statements is true of the DRG system?
   a. The DRG system considers the number of physicians within a practice and the average amount of procedures that they perform in a day.
   b. DRGs are the structural framework to the payment system of private practices.
   c. The implementation of the DRG system has caused many hospitals to increase the length of inpatient stays.
   d. As a result of the DRG system, a hospital makes a greater profit when they use fewer resources to treat a patient.

10. What is the objective of the APC payment system?
    a. To control costs and increase efficiencies for physician outpatient services
    b. To control costs and increase efficiencies for hospital outpatient services
    c. To provide payment based solely on the quality of care
    d. To provide payment based solely on the quantity of care

11. Which claim form is most commonly used in hospitals?
    a. UB-04
    b. AMA-71
    c. CMS-1500
    d. UB-92

12. Given the following information, what diagnosis code(s) should be reported?

    Discharge Summary:
    Patient was admitted 2 days ago with complaints of left upper abdominal pain, nausea, and vomiting. Physical exam and CT scans appear to be normal. Probable ischemic bowel disease vs. acute pancreatitis. Supportive treatment given. Advised rest and adequate fluid intake. Patient okay to discharge. Advised to return if pain becomes more widespread or if stools appear bloody.

    a. K55.059, K85.90
    b. R10.12, R11.2
    c. K55.059, K85.90, R10.12, R11.2
    d. K55.059

13. A patient is seen in an outpatient setting and is equally treated for two conditions. Which condition should be reported first on the claim?
    a. The condition that has the greater chance of mortality should be reported first.
    b. The condition that the patient complains about the most should be reported first.
    c. The condition with the higher reimbursement rate should be reported first.
    d. Either condition may be sequenced first.

14. Which CPT code(s) accurately describe the following ultrasound results?
    **Transabdominal U/S at 11w 2d gestation:**
    Single fetus
    Fetal HR: 143 bpm
    CRL: 51 mm
    BPD: 15.2 mm
    NT measurement obtained through transvaginal U/S: 3.5 mm
    Nasal bone present
    Placenta and amniotic fluid WNL
    Right ovary seen with corpus luteum cyst measuring 49×41×46 mm—will monitor
    a. 76818, 76819
    b. 76818
    c. 76801, 76813
    d. 76801, 76817

15. A patient is admitted for acute on chronic stage 4 kidney failure. The patient also has type 2 diabetes controlled by metformin. What ICD-10-CM codes should be assigned?
    a. N17.9, N18.4, E11.9, Z79.84
    b. N18.4, N17.9, E11.9, Z79.84
    c. N17.9, E11.22, N18.4, Z79.84
    d. E11.22, N18.4, N17.9, Z79.84

16. A physician documents that a patient has hypertension, diabetes managed with insulin, and chronic kidney disease stage 2. The CAC system generates I10, E13.9, N18.2, and Z79.4. What should be reported instead?
    a. E13.22, N18.2, I10, Z79.4
    b. E11.22, N18.2, I10, Z79.4
    c. I12.9, E11.22, N18.2, Z79.4
    d. I12.9, N18.2, E11.9, Z79.4

17. Which of the following documents can be reviewed to determine areas of audits and evaluations for the current fiscal year?
    a. CDC Coding Draft
    b. OIG Work Plan
    c. AHIMA Target Program
    d. CMS Letter of Intent

18. In the absence of state guidance, how long after the most recent encounter does AHIMA recommend that a medical practice or hospital retain confidential medical records?

   a. 2 years
   b. 5 years
   c. 7 years
   d. 10 years

19. A physician first performs a diagnostic transoral esophagoscopy on a patient, followed by a colonoscopy. If the esophagoscopy has a relative value unit of 8.06 and the colonoscopy has a relative value unit of 10.32, how should these services be reported?

   a. 43200, 45378
   b. 43200
   c. 45378, 43200-51
   d. 45378, 43200-59

20. Which type of query is documented below?

   The patient was admitted with sepsis and was temporarily put on ventilator support due to respiratory failure. Can your diagnosis of sepsis be further specified as with septic shock?

   a. Compliant multiple-choice query
   b. Noncompliant multiple-choice query
   c. Compliant yes/no query
   d. Noncompliant yes/no query

21. Which of the following factors is NOT considered when the DRG system calculates payment?

   a. Principal procedure
   b. Principal diagnosis
   c. Medical education costs
   d. Hospital demographics

22. Where can a coder find guidance on how to properly assign and report codes consistent with code set conventions, rules, and guidelines?

   a. AHA
   b. HIM Practice Excellence
   c. AHIMA Code of Ethics
   d. UHDDS

23. Which CPT code is NOT covered under Medicare Part B?

   a. G0438
   b. 99222
   c. 99282
   d. G0008

### 24. In general, most medical record encounters will include which of the following components?

a. Cardiology report
b. Review of systems
c. Pathology results
d. Discharge summary

### 25. What is the primary purpose of the risk adjustment model?

a. To inform the CDC of potential health threats or pandemics
b. To explain where government funds are being allocated
c. To assess the amount of risk being taken to insure an individual
d. To predict healthcare costs of certain groups of patients enrolled in Medicare Advantage plans

### 26. How long does HIPAA allow physicians to fulfill a medical record request?

a. 24 hours
b. 15 days
c. 30 days
d. 45 days

### 27. Which ICD-10-CM codes should be reported for the following physician's note?

62-year-old male patient being seen for follow-up on pneumonia. Completed course of azithromycin and is exhibiting no symptoms. Patient also has a history of leg pain. Patient to follow up in 6 months for annual wellness check.

a. Z09, Z87.01, Z87.39
b. Z09, Z87.01
c. J18.9, Z87.39, Z09
d. J18.9, Z09

### 28. A covered entity may require that an individual do which of the following in order to obtain access to their personal medical records?

a. Provide a written request.
b. Provide proof of identity in person.
c. Use a web portal to submit their request.
d. Submit a request by mail.

### 29. Which of the following is the claim form most commonly used in private practices?

a. UB-04
b. AMA-71
c. CMS-1500
d. UB-92

### 30. Which of the following items is NOT reviewed during a risk adjustment data validation audit?

a. Whether the record is legible
b. If there is a diagnosis on record
c. If the provider type is an MD
d. Whether the diagnosis supports an HCC

**31. NCDs and LCDs are released by which of the following?**
   a. The Office of Inspector General
   b. The Centers for Medicare & Medicaid Services
   c. The Centers for Control and Prevention
   d. The American Medical Association

**32. A patient is admitted to the hospital due to a chemical burn caused by paint thinner. The physician diagnoses the patient with second- and third-degree burns on the right hand. The physician follows up with the patient 3 days later and concludes that an infection has developed on the right hand as a result of the burn. The physician reports the injury as subsequent treatment. What should be reported instead?**
   a. L08.9, T23.201S, T23.361S, T23.301S, T54.2X4A
   b. T23.201A, T23.361A, T23.301A, T54.2X4A, L08.9
   c. T23.701A, T54.2X1A, L08.9
   d. L08.9, T23.701S, T54.2X1S

**33. Which of the following is a quality measurement tool used to report the quality of care delivered in a home health setting?**
   a. CQM
   b. HHA
   c. OASIS
   d. MDS

**34. A 72-year-old female patient is seen in the emergency room due to uncontrolled seizures. An on-call neurologist performs an expanded problem-focused history and exam, and admits the patient. The patient is given fosphenytoin through an IV drip, and a head CT is ordered to evaluate for any recent injuries. CPT code 99285 is automatically generated for this encounter. Which of the following CPT codes should be reported instead?**
   a. 99221
   b. 99283
   c. 99232
   d. 99222

**35. Which of the following errors would be flagged in a quantitative analysis of a medical record?**
   a. Copying and pasting
   b. Missing attestation
   c. Incomplete family history
   d. Contraindication in documentation

**36. The AHIMA Standards of Ethical Coding encourage which of the following actions?**
   a. Altering information within a health record to match the reported CPT code
   b. Assigning diagnosis codes reported on a previous encounter for a current encounter
   c. Taking measures to expose the negligent conduct of coworkers
   d. Using a different encounter within a patient's health record to generate a physician query

37. If a patient is admitted to the hospital with two conditions that both meet the criteria of principal diagnosis, which condition should be reported first on the claim?
    a. The condition that has the greater chance of mortality
    b. The condition that the patient complains about the most
    c. The condition with the higher reimbursement rate
    d. Either condition

38. Which element is missing in the following documented history of present illness?
    > Patient is seen in the ER complaining of sharp abdominal pains that began last night after eating at a new restaurant.
    a. Timing
    b. Duration
    c. Context
    d. Quality

39. A 59-year-old male is admitted with second- and third-degree burns to the face and third-degree burns to the chest after catching on fire while grilling. He also has extensive scarring on his right forearm due to a second-degree burn from several years ago. How should this be coded?
    a. T20.30XA, T21.31XA, X03.0XXA, L90.5, T22.219S, Y93.G2
    b. T20.30XA, T21.31XA, X03.0XXA, Z87.828, Y93.G2
    c. T20.30XA, T20.20XA, T21.31XA, X03.0XXA, Z87.828, Y93.G2
    d. T20.30XA, T20.20XA, T21.31XA, X03.0XXA, L90.5, T22.219S, Y93.G2

40. Which of the following is a commonly used encoder?
    a. Allscripts
    b. Cerner
    c. Epic
    d. 3M

41. Which of the following would be flagged in a qualitative analysis of a medical record?
    a. Missing attestation
    b. Unsigned documentation
    c. Copying and pasting
    d. Incomplete family history

42. A patient is seen in the emergency room complaining of chest pain. The physician performs a 12-lead ECG. How should this be coded?
    a. 99282-59, 93005
    b. 99282, 93005-59
    c. 99282-25, 93005
    d. 99282, 93005-25

43. Which of the following is NOT considered a valid exception to information blocking?
    a. Content
    b. Fees
    c. Security
    d. Time

44. Which of the following terms represents all of the HCCs submitted for a member in an entire calendar year?
   a. Risk adjustment performance
   b. Financial risk management
   c. Risk adjustment factor score
   d. Inherent risk measurement

45. Why is it important for physicians to adhere to the same coding rules and conventions found in the CPT, HCPCS, and ICD-10 manuals?
   a. In order to receive optimal reimbursement rates
   b. So an insurance company can receive, process, and issue payment within a 15-day time frame
   c. To obtain consistent data that will assist in tracking public health and to measure quality and safety practices
   d. To ensure that patients receive the same high standard of care despite the location it is rendered in

46. Which of the following diagnosis codes can only be first-listed as the primary reason for an encounter?
   a. Z37.2
   b. Z75.1
   c. Z74.2
   d. Z52.11

47. Why are OPPS status indicators assigned to procedure codes?
   a. To indicate how or if a service or supply will get reimbursed
   b. To indicate when a service or supply will get reimbursed
   c. To indicate who will reimburse a service or supply
   d. To indicate whether the physician or the hospital will receive the reimbursement

48. Which of the following is NOT an available option to look up LCDs and NCDs?
   a. Name of the procedure
   b. CPT code
   c. Clinical area
   d. Cost bracket

49. What is the purpose of a master patient index?
   a. To collectively review a patient's medical health record across a network of facilities
   b. To store patient identifiers and demographic information across a network of facilities
   c. To track the demographic information of patients seen on a particular day
   d. To locate the phone numbers of patients who have not yet confirmed their appointments

50. Which CMS payment scheme is used to award bonuses to top-performing hospitals and penalize low-performing hospitals by evaluating patient experience, outcomes, processes, and utilization?
   a. Common compensation system
   b. Fee-for-service
   c. Documentation improvement incentive
   d. Pay-for-performance

51. When determining an outpatient E/M level based on time, which of the following is true?
    a. Time spent reviewing a medical record prior to a visit may be counted.
    b. Time can be used to determine the level of an E/M only if 50% or more of that time was spent counseling and coordinating patient care.
    c. Only face-to-face time may be counted.
    d. Time spent by clinical staff in prepping a patient and delivering results may be counted.

52. A patient who has previously tested positive for HIV is admitted to the hospital for varicella-zoster virus. How should this be reported on the claim?
    a. B01.9
    b. B01.9, B20
    c. B01.9, Z21
    d. B20, B01.9

53. A diagnostic arthroscopy is performed on bilateral elbows. If the NCCI MUE value for CPT code 29830 is 1, how should the physician report the service?
    a. 29830-RT, 29830-LT-51
    b. 29830-RT, 29830-LT-59
    c. 29830-50
    d. 29830

54. An adult patient is seen for an annual wellness visit. The patient also has a medical history of COPD, hypertension, and anemia. What diagnoses should be reported for this encounter?
    a. Z00.01
    b. Z00.00
    c. Z00.01, J44.9, I10, D64.9
    d. Z00.00, J44.9, I10, D64.9

55. What resources are available for healthcare staff to determine best practices on confidentiality, privacy, and security?
    a. HIPAA, HHS, OCR, AMA
    b. WHO, AAPC, AHIMA
    c. AMA, CMS, AAPC
    d. HHS, OCR, FTC, ONC

56. Which of the following components of the EHR contains a chronological summary of the patient's conditions and treatments?
    a. Clinical observations
    b. Consultation reports
    c. Patient instructions
    d. Medical history

57. A patient is seen at 36 weeks and 6 days of gestation for a follow-up visit on her diabetes, for which she has been taking insulin for several years. Her blood sugar logs are normal and show that she has been adhering to her diet and medication regimen. How should this be reported?
   a. E08.9, Z79.4, Z3A.37
   b. O24.113, E11.9, Z79.4, Z3A.36
   c. O24.313, Z79.4, Z3A.36
   d. O24.414, Z3A.37

58. A patient with a second-degree heart block receives a pacemaker. The patient returns 3 days later with complaints of shortness of breath and is found to have a large intracardiac thrombus, which requires surgical intervention. If the same physician who performed the first procedure also performs the second, which modifier should be appended to the second procedure?
   a. 24
   b. 79
   c. 58
   d. 78

59. Which NCCI edit prevents payment from being issued on services on the same date that should NOT be reported together?
   a. MUE
   b. AOC
   c. AIF
   d. PTP

60. Which of the following laws require hospitals to publicly post the costs of their items and services?
   a. The HI-TECH Act
   b. Anti-Kickback Law
   c. Hospital Price Transparency Rule
   d. Stark Law

61. What is the purpose of a qualitative audit?
   a. To ensure adherence to clinical practice guidelines
   b. To assess documentation completeness
   c. To measure financial loss due to incomplete documentation
   d. To contract a physician with a private insurance carrier

62. Which organization is responsible for maintaining the CPT code set?
   a. AMA
   b. AHIMA
   c. Medical Library Association
   d. CMS

63. What are the four components of a practice management system?
   a. Reporting, scheduling, managing, submitting
   b. Scheduling, billing, storing, and reporting
   c. Billing, storing, tracking, managing
   d. Storing, reporting, processing, tracking

64. In which of the following scenarios should a coder query the physician?
   a. A physician diagnoses a patient with "borderline hypertension" at the time of inpatient discharge.
   b. A patient is evaluated for leg pain, but the physician does not indicate which side.
   c. A patient is diagnosed with acute renal insufficiency on admission, acute kidney failure during a consultation, and decreased urine output on the discharge summary.
   d. A physician documents +HIV, but there is no positive serology on file.

65. What is one objective of HIPAA?
   a. To prevent employment records from being released without prior authorization
   b. To protect the PHI of a patient
   c. To encourage healthcare providers to collaborate
   d. To provide a resource to which persons can file a complaint

66. When a teaching physician reports care rendered by a resident under the primary care exception, what modifier should be appended to the E/M code?
   a. GE
   b. GC
   c. FX
   d. FY

67. An urgent care facility performs an x-ray on a patient's thoracic spine. An independent physician reads the images. What should the physician report to the insurance carrier?
   a. 72070-TC
   b. 72070-26
   c. 72070-52
   d. 72070

68. Which of the following elements should NOT be included in the MPI?
   a. Social security number
   b. Address
   c. Resident disposition
   d. Principal diagnosis code

69. Which of the following is a performance-based measurement that aims to improve the quality, timeliness, and efficacy of healthcare?
   a. Clinical utility progress
   b. Evidence-based practice
   c. Patient-reported outcomes
   d. Clinical quality measures

**70.** A patient is admitted to inpatient hospital care and discharged 7 hours later on the next calendar day. Which CPT code should be submitted to the insurance carrier for the services rendered on the second day?

    a. 99218
    b. 99238
    c. 99221
    d. 99234

**71.** What is the purpose of a quantitative audit?

    a. To ensure adherence to clinical practice guidelines
    b. To contract a physician with a private insurance carrier
    c. To measure financial loss due to incomplete documentation
    d. To assess medical record authenticity and completeness

**72.** What specific benefit is associated with accurate coding of comorbidities?

    a. To predict risk and associated healthcare costs
    b. To educate healthcare staff
    c. To rectify conflicting documentation
    d. To optimize patient outcomes

**73.** Which of the following is NOT included in the intended objectives of the 21st Century Cures Act Final Rule?

    a. To exchange and obtain electronic health information through online portals
    b. To encourage patients and caregivers to engage in the management of their own health
    c. To block hackers from installing ransomware in hospital computer systems
    d. To promote implementation and application of an electronic medical record system among physicians and healthcare facilities who do not currently have one

**74.** According to Medicare, what is the maximum allowed timeframe for a physician to complete a medical record after a patient has been seen?

    a. 8–12 hours
    b. 12–24 hours
    c. 24–48 hours
    d. 48–72 hours

**75.** An established patient is being seen in an outpatient setting for COVID-19 complicated by pneumonia. The history of present illness is problem focused, the examination is expanded problem focused, and the medical decision making (MDM) level is moderate. How should the visit be leveled?

    a. 99212
    b. 99213
    c. 99214
    d. 99215

76. Based on the health record and documentation of a patient encounter, the electronic health system generates CPT code 99242. What is needed in order to report this code to an insurance carrier?
    a. A request from a healthcare professional
    b. A chronic illness
    c. Prior approval from the insurance carrier
    d. A written request from the patient's family

77. A 72-year-old male patient with prostate cancer is admitted for anemia associated with an adverse effect of radiotherapy. How should this be reported?
    a. D64.89, C61, T45.1X5A
    b. C61, D64.89, T45.1X5A
    c. C61, D64.89, Y84.2
    d. D64.89, C61, Y84.2

78. Which type of query is documented below?

    Can you provide a diagnosis based on the following physical findings of the patient?
    RLQ pain
    Temperature: 100.3 °F
    Urine nitrate test +

    a. Compliant open-ended query
    b. Noncompliant open-ended query
    c. Compliant yes/no query
    d. Noncompliant yes/no query

79. Which of the following types of claim denial describes a claim being denied due to a patient being covered by a different payer?
    a. Prior authorization
    b. Medical necessity
    c. Exceeded the timely filing limit
    d. Coordination of benefits

80. The patient financial services (PFS) department focuses on which billing rules?
    a. The OIG Exclusions Database
    b. CPT and ICD-10-CM coding conventions
    c. NCCI edits
    d. Local medical review policies and national coverage determinations

81. A patient's shoulder joint and knee joint were aspirated in the same session and by the same physician. If the NCCI PTP edit for these CPT codes is 1, how should the services be reported?
    a. 20610, 20610
    b. 20610, 20610-59
    c. 20610, 20610-51
    d. 20610

82. Which CPT code is NOT covered under Medicare Part A?
    a. 99291
    b. 99499
    c. 99232
    d. 99252

83. The term metastasis often refers to which of the following illnesses?
    a. Malaria
    b. Candida
    c. Gingivitis
    d. Cancer

84. A 34-year-old female patient sustained a burn injury to her face from a house fire. Two months later, a physician billed for a reconstructive burn surgery, which was denied due to being considered experimental. To obtain payment, what next step should be taken?
    a. Have the patient call the carrier
    b. Resubmit the claim with a covered procedure
    c. Submit an appeal
    d. Resubmit the procedure with a modifier

85. HIPAA-covered entities may receive PHI without a prior authorization and include which of the following?
    a. Clearinghouses, health plans, and providers
    b. Providers, health plans, and caregivers
    c. Health plans, clearinghouses, providers, and business associates
    d. Any persons included on the HIPAA disclosure form

86. A patient with uncontrolled diabetes is receiving outpatient hospice with a life expectancy of 3 weeks. The blood sugar measurement remains at 250 mg/dL, but the physician's focus is on comfort, and it is decided not to administer additional insulin. This problem is considered what level of complexity in the medical decision-making process?
    a. Minimal
    b. Low
    c. Moderate
    d. High

87. Why should a facility maintain an updated charge description master?
    a. To track claim denials and flag audit risks within a facility's billing system
    b. To ensure compliance, transparency, reimbursement, and revenue capture
    c. To track criminal cyberactivity within a hospital's EHR system
    d. To protect PHI and other private health data

88. If an insurance carrier accepts global obstetrical care only, which code should be reported for a routine prenatal visit?
    a. 59400
    b. 0502F
    c. 99213
    d. 99213-24

**89. Which of the following scenarios represents a privacy violation?**
   a. A hospital resident provides medical records to a lawyer offering his expertise for malpractice claims.
   b. A physician notifies public health officials of a positive COVID-19 result during the pandemic.
   c. A health clinic forwards medical records to a correctional facility where a patient is being held.
   d. A child suspected of being abused or neglected is reported to child protective services without permission from their legal guardian.

**90. Which of the following statements best defines encryption?**
   a. Encryption combines programming code with statistics to extract insights from data.
   b. Encryption turns text into indecipherable characters.
   c. Encryption is the process of analyzing raw data to create a statistic.
   d. Encryption is a standard protocol used to transfer electronic information between two people on the same network.

**91. Computer-assisted coding functions by automatically applying diagnosis codes based on which of the following?**
   a. The physician's clinical documentation
   b. The coder's diagnosis
   c. Documented past medical history
   d. Diagnosis codes assigned on previous claims

**92. A patient is admitted to inpatient hospital care and discharged 7 hours later on the same day. Which CPT code should be submitted to the insurance carrier?**
   a. 99218
   b. 99238
   c. 99221
   d. 99234

**93. Amniocentesis is a term associated with which specialty?**
   a. Gynecology
   b. Endocrinology
   c. Obstetrics
   d. Oncology

**94. In which scenario would the minimum necessary requirement apply?**
   a. An oncologist is requesting all medical records in the previous 5 years for treatment purposes.
   b. An employee needs access to a patient's intake form and insurance card to verify coverage.
   c. A person is requesting their own medical records.
   d. Law enforcement is requesting medical records for a child who was reported for suspicion of parental neglect.

95. Two days after a patient is seen, their lab results come back confirming the doctor's suspicion of high iron levels. How should the doctor document this?

   a. Create an entirely new note
   b. Add a late entry
   c. Make a correction
   d. Complete an addendum

96. In which of the following scenarios can a query be sent to clarify documentation that is NOT clinically supported?

   a. A patient is admitted for chest pain. The progress note on day 1 states that low-dose aspirin was administered, the progress note on day 2 shows the results of an EKG, and the discharge summary has a documented diagnosis of myocardial infarction.
   b. A patient with a past medical history of diabetes is seen for feelings of numbness in his feet. The physician's final diagnosis is diabetes.
   c. A patient is admitted with a low red blood cell count as a result of chemotherapy treatments. The physician diagnoses the patient with a history of liver cancer.
   d. A patient receives three different diagnoses by three separate doctors during the course of a hospital stay.

97. A patient's regular OB/GYN is unavailable, and an on-call physician performs an uncomplicated Cesarean delivery. The on-call physician reports CPT code 59510 in error. What can the doctor be accused of?

   a. Abuse
   b. Waste
   c. Violation of the False Claims Act
   d. Fraud

98. A female patient is seen at an outpatient clinic complaining of a sore throat. She tests positive for COVID-19 and is advised to rest and self-isolate for 14 days. Three weeks later, she returns to the clinic testing negative for COVID-19 but has developed a persistent cough. What diagnosis code(s) are associated with the second visit?

   a. Z09, R05.3, Z86.16
   b. R05.3, U09.9
   c. R05.8, Z86.16
   d. R05.8, U09.9, Z86.16

99. Which of the following will get denied based on the NCCI MUE?

   a. 44950-50
   b. 76816, 76817
   c. 21011 × 3 units
   d. 99213-25, 93000

100. HFpEF is otherwise known as which of the following conditions?

   a. High-output heart failure
   b. Diastolic heart failure
   c. Systolic heart failure
   d. Biventricular heart failure

**101.** A patient was involved in a bike and automobile accident. Who can the physician call to obtain the claim number?
   a. Employer
   b. Lawyer
   c. No-fault insurance carrier
   d. Primary care physician

**102.** The PFS department may reach out to a coder in which of the following scenarios?
   a. The date of the accident was not attached to a workers' compensation claim.
   b. A double lung transplant was billed with modifier 50 and denied for inappropriate modifier.
   c. A claim was denied due to not obtaining authorization prior to the patient encounter.
   d. A patient is seen for prescription birth control, but this service is not covered under the patient's insurance plan.

**103.** An 84-year-old female patient is seen in urgent care with complaints of weakness, dehydration, and deconditioning related to pneumonia due to COVID-19 along with advanced age. What diagnosis codes should the physician report?
   a. U07.1, J12.82, R53.1, E86.0, R53.81, R54
   b. U07.1, J12.82, E86.0, R53.81
   c. U07.1, J12.82
   d. U07.1, J12.82, R54

**104.** A 16-year-old female patient presents to the surgical room for a laparoscopic hernia repair. Due to having a urinary tract infection, the physician decides to postpone the procedure until after the patient has completed her course of antibiotics for the infection. Which ICD-10-CM and CPT codes should be assigned for this encounter?
   a. 99213, K40.90, N39.0, Z53.09
   b. 99213, Z53.09
   c. 49650-73, Z53.09
   d. 49650-53, K40.90, N39.0, Z53.09

**105.** According to HIPAA, security in the workplace includes which of the following?
   a. Administrative, physical, and technical safeguards
   b. Password changes every 90 days
   c. Individual cubicles for employees accessing PHI
   d. Password changes every 60 days

**106.** How often should a charge description master be updated?
   a. Quarterly
   b. Biannually
   c. Annually
   d. Monthly

107. A 48-year-old male patient is seen for a follow-up on his celiac disease. He also receives a gastrointestinal endoscopy due to recent complaints of nausea, vomiting, and difficulty swallowing. What CPT code(s) should the physician report for this encounter?
   a. 43235
   b. 99213-25, 43235
   c. 99213, 43235
   d. 99213, 43235-59

108. A provider documents in his assessment that a patient is obese, but the BMI extracted from the chart is consistent with morbid obesity. How should the patient's condition be reported on the claim?
   a. Morbid obesity
   b. Morbid obesity and the documented BMI
   c. Unspecified obesity
   d. Unspecified obesity and the documented BMI

109. Which of the following is an acceptable attestation to report services rendered by a resident under the care and direction of a teaching physician?
   a. "Rounded, reviewed, and agree."
   b. "I saw and evaluated the patient. Findings were discussed with the resident, and I agree with the plan as documented by the resident."
   c. "Patient seen and evaluated by the resident, and I agree with the findings and plan of care."
   d. "I discussed the case with the resident and agree with the current diagnosis. Will order MRI of the thoracic spine."

110. Which of the following CPT code pairs is a bundled charge?
   a. 31231, 30903
   b. 11102, 11103
   c. 81002, 81025
   d. 76830, 76856

111. A physician inserts a Nexplanon, a birth control implant, into a patient's arm at 9 a.m. The patient returns at 2 p.m., complaining of severe pain at the insertion site. The physician removes the Nexplanon from the patient's arm. How should the physician report the encounters?
   a. 11982, 11981-59
   b. 11981, 11982
   c. 11983
   d. 11981, 11982-51

112. What ICD-10-CM code(s) should be reported for the following note?
   Patient is seen 2 days after an appendectomy with complaints of nausea and cramping. Physical examination shows slight dehiscence at the surgical site. Advised patient that symptoms will resolve in 24 hours with rest and increased fluid intake. Dx: Ileus
   a. Z48.815
   b. K91.89, Z98.890
   c. Z09, Z87.19
   d. K91.89, Z48.815

# Answer Key and Explanations for Test #2

**1. A:** The proper disposal of confidential medical records involves the complete destruction of personally identifiable data. For paper records, this includes shredding, pulverization, incineration pulping, or transferring records to a destruction or disposal vendor. For electronic records, this includes the physical destruction of the computer hard drive or other practices that overwrite protected health information (PHI), such as digital sanitation or degaussing. When disposing of confidential medical records, a log should be kept containing minimal demographic information, along with the date, method of destruction, and any witnesses present at the time of disposal. When using a destruction or disposal vendor, a certificate of destruction should be issued.

**2. A:** Because medical decision making is the driving force for determining the level of service, ancillary staff may contribute to the documentation of a medical record. However, ICD-10-CM guidelines state that "the assignment of a diagnosis code is based only on the provider's diagnostic statement." There are some exceptions, including BMI, depth or stage of an ulcer, Glasgow Coma Scale, National Institutes of Health Stroke Scale, social determinants of health (SDOH), laterality, blood alcohol level, and an underimmunzation status. To report these secondary diagnoses, the provider would need to document the associated condition. In this scenario, to report the patient's BMI, the provider would have had to indicate that the patient was overweight or obese.

**3. B:** According to the AHIMA Standards of Ethical Coding, diagnosis and procedure codes must be reported in a way that most accurately represents the care rendered. In this scenario, by excluding birth control from the claim, a coding professional is intentionally omitting information in order to receive reimbursement from the insurance carrier. Although sending a query to a physician to confirm a suspected condition, using a search engine to locate a diagnosis code, and providing unsolicited advice to a physician are not advantageous actions, they are not considered violations of the AHIMA Standards of Ethical Coding.

**4. A:** When abstracting data from a health record, obtaining an accurate and specific diagnosis is essential, because it affects reimbursement rates and resource utilization. In this scenario, postprocedural hypothyroidism (E89.0), acute schizophrenia (F20.9), and tineas corporis (B35.4) are the most specific descriptors for their category of diseases. On the other hand, chronic kidney disease (CKD) is an illness that presents itself in six stages. By reporting CKD unspecified, as opposed to its specific stage, a facility cuts their reimbursement rate by almost 50%.

**5. B:** The HIPAA Privacy Rule is a federal law established in 1996 to protect a patient's health information from being disclosed without their consent. However, the HIPAA Privacy Rule does allow a covered entity, including health plans, clearinghouses, and healthcare providers, to release health information for purposes of obtaining and releasing eligibility, authorizations, payment, and continuing care. In this scenario, the HIPAA Privacy Rule allows one physician to request records from another physician without obtaining an authorization from the patient because it involves continuity of care.

**6. D:** In an outpatient setting, if a diagnosis is listed as "possible," "probable," "suspected," "likely," "concern for," or "questionable," this should not be reported. Only the signs and symptoms should be reported in lieu of the uncertain diagnosis. In this scenario, because a gastrointestinal hemorrhage is only suspected, the diagnosis of melena (K92.1) and dark, tarry stool (R19.5) should be coded. However, the diagnosis code K92.1 contains an "excludes 1" marker associated with diagnosis code R19.5, indicating that these codes should never be used at the same time. Therefore, only melena (K92.1) should be coded for this encounter.

**7. A:** A resection is the removal of an organ or tissue from the body. Therefore, a resection performed on the large bowel would involve the full or partial removal of the cecum, colon, rectum, or anal canal. In this scenario, the procedure is a partial resection, otherwise known as a colectomy. In the CPT Index, search "colectomy" followed by "partial" to arrive at code 44140 (colectomy, partial; with anastomosis). Anastomosis is a surgical connection between the two parts of the intestine made with either staples or sutures and is considered a necessary part of this procedure.

**8. A:** If an arthroscopy is converted to an open procedure, only report the open procedure. Additionally, there is an "excludes" note attached to CPT code 29827 (arthroscopy, shoulder, surgical; with rotator cuff repair), indicating that CPT codes 23410 (repair of ruptured musculotendinous cuff, open; acute) and 23412 (repair of ruptured musculotendinous cuff, open; chronic) are more appropriate codes if such a service took place.

**9. D:** In general, prior to 1983, hospitals would treat patients over a longer span of time, use unnecessary supplies, and perform as many procedures as possible to increase their profit margin. However, when the diagnosis-related group (DRG) system was implemented, hospitals were no longer paid for each charge they reported; rather, they were paid based on other factors relating to the patient (i.e., age, sex, disabilities), their condition(s), and the expected treatment protocols. As a result, it forced hospitals to analyze how to treat their patients most effectively and efficiently, because spending less time and resources resulted in a higher profit.

**10. B:** The ambulatory payment classification (APC) system is used by Medicare to control costs and increase the efficiency of care for hospital outpatient services. Rather than paying hospitals for multiple itemized charges, Medicare uses the APC system to group procedures that are clinically similar (i.e., the same body system) and use similar resources (i.e., staff, procedure time, medical supplies, etc.) to issue a predetermined payment. For example, CPT codes 20251 (biopsy, vertebral body, open) and 20690 (application of uniplane, unilateral, external fixation system) both fall under APC grouping 5114, level 4. Therefore, although these procedures may be performed at different times and on different patients, the hospital outpatient facility would receive the same reimbursement rate for both.

**11. A:** The UB-04 Form, also known as the CMS-1450 Form, replaces the UB-92 Form and is used by hospitals and outpatient facilities to report services covered under Medicare Part A, which include surgeries, radiology and laboratory services, and inpatient therapies. Additionally, if a physician from a private practice uses the space and resources of a hospital or outpatient facility to perform a procedure, the UB-04 Form may be submitted to report such a use. The UB-04 Form may be submitted electronically or through the mail on paper.

**12. A:** In an inpatient setting, if a diagnosis is listed as "possible," "probable," "suspected," "likely," "concern for," or "questionable," this should be reported if documented at the time of discharge. Signs and symptoms should not be reported in lieu of the uncertain diagnosis. In this scenario, because ischemic bowel disease and acute pancreatitis are suspected, they both should be reported. Exceptions to this rule are diagnoses of HIV/AIDS, identified influenza, and Zika virus, which require confirmation.

**13. D:** In an outpatient setting, the primary condition or illness that is most responsible for the encounter is termed as the first-listed diagnosis. When a patient is seen in an outpatient setting and is equally treated for two conditions that meet the definition of first-listed diagnosis, either condition may be sequenced first, unless the ICD-10 guidelines state otherwise for the specific conditions being reported.

**14. C:** Ultrasounds are reported based on the imaging technique used, gestational age of the fetus, and fetal and/or maternal structures documented. To locate an ultrasound code, refer to the CPT Coding Expert Index and search "ultrasound." The term "fetus" will direct you to CPT codes 76818 and 76819, but the term "pregnant uterus" will direct you to CPT codes 76801–76817. In this scenario, the patient is in her first trimester, the imaging technique used was a transabdominal approach, and both fetal and maternal structures were documented. Therefore, the code that accurately describes the procedure performed is 76801 (ultrasound, pregnant uterus, real time with image documentation, fetal and maternal evaluation, first trimester, transabdominal approach, single or first gestation). Additionally, NT is an abbreviation for nuchal translucency, and it is reported with CPT code 76813 (ultrasound, pregnant uterus, real time with image documentation, first trimester fetal nuchal translucency measurement, transabdominal or transvaginal approach, single or first gestation).

**15. C:** When coding the same condition, always sequence the acute diagnosis, followed by the chronic diagnosis. When the word "with" appears in a code title, a causal relationship between the two diagnoses can be assumed, even when the physician's documentation does not explicitly link them. In this scenario, acute kidney failure (N17.9) would be sequenced first. Then, because ICD-10-CM guidelines advise that any associated diabetic chronic kidney disease should be reported before the chronic kidney disease, E11.22 would be the secondary code, followed by N18.4, and the means by which the diabetes is controlled (Z79.–) is reported last.

**16. C:** Even with CAC automatically documenting and generating diagnosis codes based on physician documentation, coding professionals are still needed to validate, amend, and submit codes. This is because CAC often picks up on a diagnosis without considering the entirety of a record or the ICD-10 guidelines. In this scenario, the CAC was correct in that the patient has hypertension, diabetes with long-term insulin use, and chronic kidney disease stage 2, but it does not recognize that hypertension and diabetes have a causal relationship to chronic kidney disease. When a coding professional reviews the charges that were posted automatically, they can manually correct these assignments.

**17. B:** The Office of Inspector General (OIG) works under the direction of the US Department of Health and Human Services (HHS) and aims to detect fraud, waste, and abuse within the Centers for Medicare & Medicaid Services (CMS). Each fiscal year, the OIG creates what is known as the Work Plan, which identifies and targets specific issues within a medical record or healthcare setting. By regularly reviewing the OIG Work Plan, coders can be alert to any documentation patterns or physician behaviors that put their organization at risk for future audits, payment adjustments, or recoupments.

**18. D:** Although there are currently no federal regulations outlining the length of time that a medical practice or hospital must retain confidential medical records, healthcare physicians and facilities should consult their local state requirements. In the absence of state guidance, AHIMA recommends that an adult medical record be retained for 10 years after the most recent encounter and 10 years following a child's 18th birthday. For example, California requires that medical records be retained for 10 years after a patient's most recent encounter, whereas New York only requires a retention period of 6 years.

**19. C:** Modifier 51 is needed when multiple procedures are performed in the same session that routinely occur together. However, when modifier 51 is appended, a multiple procedure payment reduction is often applied, which may deduct up to 50% of the reimbursement rate. Because of this high reduction in payment, it is important to apply modifier 51 to the procedure with the lowest amount of relative value units, which are a measure of value that determine how much a physician or facility will be reimbursed for services rendered.

**20. D:** This is a noncompliant yes/no query. A yes/no query is one in which the physician can respond with either a yes or a no. Although it is true that sepsis can lead to organ failure and is termed as septic shock, the query is noncompliant because it leads the physician to a specific diagnosis. A more appropriate form of query for this scenario would be an open-ended query or a multiple-choice query, which would allow the physician to choose which diagnosis is applicable to the patient's condition.

**21. C:** Usually, DRG assignment is based on the principal diagnosis, but in some cases, the principal diagnosis alone does not accurately reflect the severity of an illness or the resources that were used. In these cases, the DRG assignment may be based on the procedures performed. For example, a patient with liver disease is admitted to the hospital for a liver transplant. In this scenario, the principal diagnosis of liver disease would not reimburse the hospital for the costs incurred for performing a liver transplant and all associated care. When determining payment, the DRG system will also consider the demographic location of the hospital. For example, the costs of equipment and staff are higher in New York City than in Wichita, Kansas. As a result, the same procedure can be performed in either city, but a New York City hospital would receive a higher reimbursement.

**22. C:** Coders can access the AHIMA Code of Ethics to find guidance on how to properly assign and report codes consistent with code set conventions, rules, and guidelines. It also includes principles on how to query a physician, reveals in what instances it would be appropriate to do so, and provides a framework for professional behavior in order to improve the quality of care given in any healthcare setting.

**23. B:** Medicare Part B provides patients with coverage on outpatient services such as annual wellness exams (G0438–G0439), vaccine administrations (G0008–G0010), and emergency room encounters (99281–99285). Any type of hospital or inpatient admission (99220–99233) and care are covered and should be billed to Medicare Part A. Medicare Part D covers prescription drugs. Medicare Part C plans, otherwise known as Medicare Advantage Plans, provide additional coverage not otherwise available under Part B plans.

**24. B:** Although documentation methods vary for each physician, the medical record for an encounter will generally begin with the patient's chief complaint, which is the primary reason for the encounter. Following that would be a patient's past, social, and family history. This information may or may not be contained in separate tabs in an electronic medical record. Next may be a review of systems, in which the patient has the opportunity to confirm or deny signs and symptoms pertaining to their different body systems. Next is a physical exam, usually focused around the patient's chief complaint. Once the physician has collected an intake from the patient and examined the patient, it is then time to make a diagnosis and a plan of how to address the patient's concerns.

**25. D:** The primary purpose of the risk adjustment model is to predict healthcare costs of patients enrolled in Medicare Advantage plans. The risk adjustment model is created based on the CMS hierarchical condition category (HCC) model, which categorizes patients with specific diseases or conditions that have a similar long-term cost burden. Medicare then reviews this information to provide a capitation payment to the health plan. This capitation payment not only relieves the health plan of some of the financial burden, but it also provides an incentive to enroll patients with chronic and/or serious health conditions.

**26. C:** HIPAA allows physicians 30 calendar days to fulfill a medical record request, but a single extension of 30 days may be allowed if there are extenuating circumstances that prevent the records from being given to the person(s) requesting them. Although most physicians can fulfill this request within hours or days, others take more time to locate the records, select the requested information, review the documents, and then prepare the records to be sent (e.g., electronically, by mail, or by fax).

**27. B:** A follow-up code (Z08–Z09, Z39) is used to indicate that an illness was treated and no longer exists. Follow-up codes are coded first and require that a history code be added to elaborate on the condition that was treated, but no longer exists. Additionally, ICD-10-CM guidelines state that history codes (categories Z80–Z87) may be reported only if the condition or family history has an impact on the current care plan or if it influences the course of treatment. In this scenario, Z09 would be coded as primary, followed by Z87.01 (personal history of pneumonia). The code Z87.39 (personal history of other diseases of the musculoskeletal system) would not be used because it has no impact on the current or future treatment plan or the current health of the patient.

**28. A:** The HIPAA Privacy Rule dictates that a covered entity may require that an individual provide a written request to obtain access to their medical records. This may be in the form of an electronic request, such as by email or through a web portal, or it may be a paper request. The Privacy Rule does not allow covered entities to require proof of identity in person, use a web portal, or mail a request. These options are considered unreasonable because a person may be homebound or may not have access to the internet, or these restrictions could can cause an unnecessary delay in retrieving patients' medical records.

**29. C:** The CMS-1500 Form, also known as the HCFA form, is used by private practices and physicians to report services covered under Medicare Part B, including doctor visits and home health services. Additionally, if a physician from a private practice uses a hospital or outpatient surgical center to perform a procedure, the physician would bill services only on the CMS-1500 Form. This form may be submitted electronically or through the mail on paper.

**30. C:** Risk adjustment data validation audits are performed by CMS annually and require medical records to meet certain documentation standards to avoid a payment adjustment or total recoupment. Knowing in advance what will be reviewed can assist coders in being aware of missing items prior to an audit request. According to ICD-10-CM, these items include:

- The record must be for the correct enrollee.
- The record must be from the correct calendar year for the payment year being audited.
- The record must be legible.
- The date of service must be present on the records and is for a face-to-face visit.
- The record must be from a valid provider type.
- Valid credentials and/or a valid physician specialty must be documented on the record.
- The record must contain a signature from an acceptable type of physician.
- There must be a diagnosis on the record.
- The diagnosis must support an HCC.
- The diagnosis must support the submitted HCC.

**31. B:** Local coverage determinations (LCDs) and national coverage ceterminations (NCDs) are released by CMS. LCDs determine coverage for certain services based on medical necessity and change in each contracted region. NCDs identify coverage for certain services that are applicable to all members nationwide. LCDs and NCDs are updated on a quarterly basis with the release of coding additions and revisions.

**32. C:** A burn caused by a chemical would be considered a corrosion, because it is not caused by heat, electricity, or radiation. Additionally, when multiple burns on the same anatomic location and laterality are being treated, only the diagnosis with the highest degree of burn recorded should be reported. In this scenario, that would be the third-degree burns on the right hand. Additionally, although the skin infection is a sequela, the seventh character in the corrosion code would remain "A" and would be sequenced first to indicate that the patient is still receiving active treatment for the reason of admission.

**33. C:** The home health Outcome and Assessment Information Set (OASIS) is a quality measurement tool used to report and improve the quality of care delivered to Medicare and Medicaid patients in the home health setting. The data collected include observation, interviews with the patient and other associated healthcare providers, and review of related medical records. Based on this information, a home health agency will develop and implement a quality improvement plan. Assessments are performed at the start of care followed by a reassessment every 60 days and again at the patient's death, discharge, or transfer to an inpatient facility. A home health agency is required to submit the data to CMS within 30 days of their collection.

**34. C:** CPT codes 99221–99223 (initial hospital care, per day, for E/M of a patient) are reported at the time of hospital admission by the physician doing the admitting. However, in order to report these codes, the physician must document at a minimum a detailed history, a detailed exam, and a straightforward MDM process. When the documentation does not meet these standards, CMS has advised physicians to report CPT codes 99231–99233 (subsequent hospital care, per day, for E/M of a patient). In this scenario, the physician documented a problem-focused history and exam. The MDM process is considered moderate based on the uncertainty of the prognosis and the administration of the fosphenytoin. Therefore, the CPT code that should be reported is 99232.

**35. B:** A missing attestation would be flagged in a quantitative analysis of a medical record because it is part of the physician's authentication of what was done. An attestation is written proof that a teaching physician has independently evaluated the patient or was physically present for the critical portions of an exam rendered by a resident and takes part in the management of care.

**36. C:** The AHIMA Standards of Ethical Coding is a set of guidelines and expectations set forth to ensure that moral decision-making, conduct, and activities are performed within the healthcare setting. This includes taking immediate action to discourage, prevent, expose, and correct unethical conduct if observed in the workplace. These guidelines apply not only to coding professionals, but also to auditors, educators, students, managers, and clinical documentation improvement professionals. All employees must work together to create a workplace environment that fosters honesty and adherence to local laws and government regulations.

**37. D:** The Uniform Hospital Discharge Data Set (UHDDS) defines a principal diagnosis as the condition or illness that is most responsible for the reason of admission into the hospital for care. When a patient is admitted to the hospital with two conditions that equally meet the criteria of principal diagnosis, either condition may be sequenced first, unless the ICD-10 guidelines state otherwise for the specific conditions being reported.

**38. A:** The elements included in a history of present illness are location (i.e., where the problem occurs), timing (i.e., how often it occurs), modifying factors (i.e., what has been done to help the problem), severity (being rated on a scale of 1–10), duration (i.e., when the problem began), associated signs and/or symptoms (i.e., anything else that is unusual for the patient), quality (i.e., the adjectives used to describe the problem), and context (i.e., what activity was being done when the problem began). In this scenario, how often the abdominal pain is occurring (e.g., constant or it comes and goes) is not documented. Although outpatient services no longer consider the history of present illness when determining the level of service, it is still a required component during level selection for inpatient services.

**39. A:** Burn codes are sequenced in order of most severe (third-degree burns) to least severe (first-degree burns). Additionally, when multiple burns are being treated on the same anatomical location and the same side of the body, only the burn that reflects the highest degree of severity should be reported. In this scenario, only the third-degree burns to the face (T20.30XA) and the third-degree burns to the chest (T21.31XA) are coded, followed by the agent (X03.0XXA), and the activity the patient was involved in when the injury occurred (Y93.G2). Because the physician documented the existence of a sequela of a previous burn, it should be coded as such (L90.5, T22.219S), rather than a history of healed trauma.

**40. D:** During the 1990s, encoding software was released that allowed medical coders to shift from searching through manuals to accessing just one portal to locate any HCPCS Level II, ICD-10, and CPT code. Encoding software not only serves as a tool for coding and classification, but it also provides guidance on reimbursement methodologies, clinical documentation integrity, and quality. Some of the most commonly used encoders include Encoder Pro, 3M, and AHIMA VLab.

**41. C:** Duplication or repetition in documentation, otherwise known as cloning or copying and pasting, would be flagged in a qualitative analysis of a medical record. Although some demographic information may be brought forward from an existing note, the actual history, evaluation, and plan of treatment for the patient should be originated on the date the patient was actually seen. When these aspects of the note are copied and pasted from previous dates of service, the actual author of the note and their thoughts on the patient's condition become ambiguous, which may adversely affect patient care.

**42. C:** Modifier 25 is reported to indicate that an E/M service is separately identifiable to a procedure or other service done by the same physician on the same date and may be appended only to office or outpatient services (99201–99215), emergency department services (99281–99285), critical care services (99291), and office or other outpatient consultations (99241–99245). In this scenario, an E/M is performed (99282), in addition to a 12-lead ECG (93005). Modifier 59 is used to indicate that two independent, non-E/M services are being performed on the same day.

**43. D:** There are eight exceptions to information blocking, which may prevent or delay a healthcare entity from fulfilling a request to exchange, use, or access PHI:

- Preventing harm
- Privacy
- Security
- Infeasibility
- Health information technology performance
- Content and manner
- Fees
- Licensing

**44. C:** All of the HCCs submitted for a member in an entire calendar year cumulate to a risk adjustment factor (RAF) score. For a new member enrolled in a Medicare Advantage plan for fewer than 12 months, the RAF score is calculated based on their age, sex, and current disabilities. An RAF score for a healthy, adult patient is 1.0, and the score increases when the patient sustains a severe injury and/or chronic illness. Therefore, accurate coding for patients with Medicare Advantage plans is imperative because overcoding or falsely inflating diagnoses will result in higher government funding, whereas under- or incomplete coding may result in not enough funding.

**45. C:** It is important for physicians to adhere to the same coding rules and conventions when assigning CPT, HCPCS, and ICD-10 codes for the purpose of tracking public health data and for the federal government to measure quality and safety practices. These data are collected for present and future use. However, in order for them to be reliable and accurate, the data must be consistent: The same coding rules and conventions need to be followed by everyone. Additionally, when physicians and coding professionals allow reimbursement to inappropriately influence code assignment, they put themselves and their facilities at risk for audits, fines, and healthcare exclusions.

**46. D:** Appendix D in the ICD-10-CM manual lists all of the Z codes that can only be used as the principal reason for an encounter and includes Z52.11 (skin donor, autologous). Within the ICD-10-CM, CPT, and HCPCS manuals are multiple appendices that may be used to review anatomy, coding and documentation guidelines, medically unlikely edits (MUEs), modifiers, and more.

**47. A:** The Medicare Outpatient Prospective Payment System (OPPS) status indicators are assigned to CPT and HCPCS level II codes to indicate how or if Medicare will reimburse for a service or supply in an outpatient hospital setting. For example, an ambulance transport has a status indicator of "A," meaning that it will be paid according to a fee schedule. However, anesthesia and IV supplies have a status indicator of "N," meaning that Medicare considers these as bundled into whatever procedure was performed that day. Coders should be aware of these status indicators because it not only saves time in having to report multiple unnecessary charges, but it also helps protect the hospital from being flagged for an audit due to inappropriate coding or unbundling.

**48. D:** LCDs and NCDs can be found by searching the name of a procedure, CPT code, clinical area, or document ID number or by looking at an alphabetical list of the procedures covered by Medicare. Because NCDs and LCDs are updated quarterly, general search results found on the internet should not be relied on as a tool to interpret coverage. Rather, current NCDs and LCDs can be accessed via the CMS website.

**49. B:** A master patient index (MPI) is a database that stores patient identifiers, demographic information, admission into an inpatient facility, and discharge and transfer dates from an inpatient facility across a network of healthcare facilities. This unique identifier, also known as a National Health ID number, is then linked to local identifiers issued throughout the network. An MPI plays an important role in information exchange and consolidation of patient lists within a facility's databases.

**50. D:** When abstracted data show that patients are generally satisfied with their healthcare, death rates and readmission rates are low, physicians adhere to best medical practices, and the resources are used conservatively to treat and diagnose patients, the result is a high CMS pay-for-performance score. The highest-ranking hospitals receive monetary bonuses, whereas the lowest-ranking hospitals receive a penalty in an effort to increase the quality of care and decrease costs and adverse effects.

**51. A:** Prior to 2021, time could be used to determine the level of an E/M service only when 50% or more of that time was spent counseling and coordinating patient care. However, effective January 2021, AMA and CMS proclaimed that total face-to-face and non-face-to-face time on the date of an outpatient encounter may be used to determine the level of an E/M service, including time spent reviewing a medical record prior to meeting with the patient. This time is only the physician's time and cannot be combined with time spent by the clinical staff in either prepping a patient, collecting a history intake, or delivering results.

**52. D:** According to the ICD-10 guidelines, if a patient who has previously tested positive for HIV disease is admitted to the hospital with an HIV disease-related illness, diagnosis code B20 (human immunodeficiency virus) should be listed as the principal diagnosis, followed by the HIV disease-related illness and other conditions. Diagnosis code Z21 (asymptomatic human immunodeficiency virus infection status) should not be reported in lieu of an HIV disease-related illness, even when the physician does not explicitly link the two conditions. An HIV disease-related illness can be identified by locating the HIV icon in the ICD-10 manual.

**53. C:** An MUE value of 1 indicates that a procedure can only be reported one time on the same date of service for a patient. Because CPT code 29830 (arthroscopy, elbow, diagnostic [separate procedure]) is a unilateral procedure, modifier 50 can be appended to indicate that it was performed on both elbows. Additionally, the term "separate procedure" listed in the description of the code means that the procedure is an integral part of a much bigger service but can also be carried out independently. It does not mean that the CPT code can be reported twice for a bilateral encounter.

**54. D:** Chronic obstructive pulmonary disease (J44.9), hypertension (I10), and anemia (D64.9) are all chronic systemic diseases that a patient should receive ongoing treatment for. Even when the physician does not explicitly document whether care was rendered for these conditions, they should be assigned as secondary diagnoses. Additionally, during a preventative visit, a condition would qualify as an abnormal finding if it was newly identified or if there was a change in severity of an existing chronic illness. In this scenario, the primary diagnosis would be Z00.00 (adult medical examination without abnormal findings) because there is no documented change to the chronic illnesses and no mention of a newly identified condition.

**55. D:** AHIMA recommends the following resources when trying to determine best practices for confidentiality, privacy, and security in the healthcare field:

- HHS and OCR (Office for Civil Rights), which can be accessed to understand how HIPAA rules apply and receive additional information blocking policies.
- FTC (Federal Trade Commission) provides guidance on protecting information when using apps, such as on a phone, computer, or iPad. FTC can also be used to report a privacy breach.
- ONC (Office of the National Coordinator for Health Information Technology) has tools to protect PHI on the internet.

**56. A:** An EHR system contains many components that collectively create a complete health record for an individual. This includes clinical observations that provide a chronological summary of a patient's conditions and treatments, consultation reports that document opinions and recommendations about the patient's condition by healthcare providers other than the attending physician, patient instructions that explain follow-up care, and medical history that describes a patient's past and current health status.

**57. B:** The documentation indicates that the patient has preexisting diabetes, and she has been taking insulin for several years. If the type of diabetes is not documented, always default to type 2. In this scenario, the [preexisting type 2] diabetes in a third-trimester pregnancy would be coded as O24.113. This would be followed by an additional code in category E11 to identify any manifestations and a code in category Z79 to identify an applicable long-term treatment of insulin or metformin. The weeks of gestation (Z3A.–) will always be sequenced last and refer only to full weeks. In this scenario, although the patient is almost at 37 weeks, she has only completed 36 full weeks of her pregnancy.

**58. D:** Modifier 78 is appended on a second, unplanned, but related procedure done during the postoperative period of the first procedure. In this scenario, an intracardiac thrombus was a complication that resulted in the unexpected return to the operating room during the postoperative period of an inserted pacemaker. Although similar, modifier 58 would be appended if the physician knew and/or planned a second, relatable procedure during the postoperative period. Modifier 79 is used when an unrelated procedure takes place during the postoperative period. Modifier 24 is used only on unrelated E/M services within the postoperative period. Of course, these rules apply when the same physician is billing for both services.

**59. D:** PTP (procedure-to-procedure) edits prevent payment from being issued on services on the same date that should not be reported together. Often, one procedure will get denied unless a modifier is associated with it that makes the procedure clinically appropriate. AOC (add-on code) edits ensure that another primary procedure is reported first and in conjunction with the secondary AOC. MUEs prevent payment from being issued on an excessive number of units and/or services being rendered in one day.

**60. C:** The Hospital Price Transparency Rule became effective on January 1, 2021. It requires that hospitals publicly post the costs of their items and services in either a comprehensive, machine-readable file or display them in a consumer-friendly format. The penalty for noncompliance is $300 to $5,500 per day—not to exceed $2,007,500 per year. This information allows consumers to understand and compare the costs of receiving potential care prior to going into the hospital.

**61. A:** The purpose of a qualitative audit is to review the documentation for inconsistencies and ensure adherence to clinical practice guidelines, regulations, and standards. This is especially applicable to long-term care facilities, which must qualitatively review and monitor their documentation on a patient's admission, return to the hospital, and upon discharge and/or death. On the other hand, a quantitative audit ensures that the medical record is authenticated and completed in a timely manner.

**62. A:** The American Medical Association (AMA) is responsible for maintaining and releasing the CPT code set each calendar year. AMA provides coding guidance and descriptors for current, revised, and added CPT codes; alerts coders of public health notices; contains tools to help locate specific CPT codes; and assists healthcare practices in implementing E/M changes. AHIMA encourages coders to use AMA as an official source of guidance when coding.

**63. B:** The four basic components of a practice management system are scheduling appointments; billing and collecting revenue for the practice; storing patient information; and generating reports from internal data that pertain to the revenue cycle, marketing, and productivity. A practice management system streamlines administrative tasks, increases productivity, and allows a practice to run smoothly.

**64. C:** When the documentation is not clear or is conflicting, the physician should be queried. In this scenario, the patient is diagnosed with three conditions that all relate to each other but are clinically different. The physician should be queried to identify the actual diagnosis of the patient. On the other hand, if a physician documents a "borderline" diagnosis on the inpatient discharge summary, the coder should code the condition as if it were confirmed. Additionally, if the laterality of a condition is not documented by the physician, a coder should choose a code indicating that the side is unspecified (e.g., M79.606: pain in leg, unspecified). Finally, although HIV cases are only to be coded if confirmed, ICD-10-CM's definition of confirmation only requires the provider's diagnostic statement that the condition exists and does not require a positive culture or test.

**65. B:** HIPAA was established as federal law in 1996 and has the following objectives:

- To prevent a person's PHI from being disclosed to a noncovered entity without permission
- To reduce healthcare fraud, waste, and abuse
- To provide a standard of security for retaining health information

Additionally, while HIPAA does provide details and principles of what would be considered a violation of the law, complaints go directly to the HHS website.

**66. A:** Because residents belonging to a primary care center generally provide care to the same patient demographic over the course of their training, the primary care exception allows teaching physicians in these centers to bill for some E/M services rendered by a resident, without requiring their physical presence or independent evaluation of the patient. These E/M services include CPT codes 99201–99215 (office and other outpatient visit), 99495–99496 (transitional care management), 99421–99423 (online digital E/M service), 99452 (interprofessional telephone/internet/electronic health record referral services), and 99441–99443 (telephone E/M service)—and HCPCS codes G2010 (remote evaluation of recorded video and/or images), G2012 (brief communication technology-based service), and G0402–G0439 (preventative and wellness visits). During level selection for an E/M under the primary care exception, teaching physicians may only use documented MDM—not time spent. Modifier GE should be appended to indicate that the teaching physician was not present under the primary care exception.

**67. B:** Modifiers TC and 26 are used on single CPT codes to indicate that the code being reported was split into two components. Modifier TC, otherwise known as the technical component, is used to report the cost that a hospital or facility incurred from the procedure or service taking place at its location (i.e., equipment, supplies, staff, etc.). Modifier 26 is used to obtain payment for the professional component of the service, including supervision and interpretation. In this scenario, because the physician reading the image is not employed by the urgent care facility, the physician would report 72070-26 and would receive approximately 40% of the payment and the urgent care facility would report 72070-TC and would receive the remaining 60%.

**68. D:** Although the specific content of the MPI may vary with each inpatient facility, AHIMA recommends that it contain the following basic information for patients:

- Medical record number
- Date of birth
- Name
- Gender
- Address
- Social security number
- Admission, discharge, and transfer dates
- Resident disposition

The principal diagnosis, other diagnoses, treatment, and past medical history are elements that should not be contained in the MPI because that would be a violation of HIPAA regulations.

**69. D:** Clinical quality measures (CQMs) were designed by CMS to improve the quality, efficacy, and timeliness of healthcare services rendered in a hospital. CQMs are established by reviewing administrative data, electronic clinical data, instruments/patient-reported outcome measures, medical records, patient experience surveys, and registries. These data can be obtained from paper, electronic, or digital records. Examples of conditions in which CMS has measured the quality of care rendered are asthma control, diabetes with complications, and the control of high blood pressure. CMS considers a hospital to have high-quality performance if it receives a score of 95% or higher.

**70. B:** According to CMS guidelines, if a patient is admitted for inpatient hospital care and discharged on a different calendar day, a code from CPT range 99221–99223 (initial hospital care, per day, for E/M of a patient) should be reported for the initial visit, followed by 99231–99234 (subsequent hospital care, per day, for E/M of a patient) for each subsequent date the patient is treated in an inpatient setting. When the patient is discharged on a different calendar day, even if their inpatient stay is less than 8 hours, CPT code 99238–99239 (hospital discharge day management) should be reported.

**71. D:** A quantitative audit is performed to confirm that medical records are authenticated and completed in a timely manner. On the other hand, a qualitative audit is performed to review for documentation inconsistencies and to ensure adherence to clinical practice guidelines, regulations, and standards.

**72. A:** A comorbidity occurs when a patient has two or more unrelated diseases or disorders occurring at the same time. Researchers and health insurance plans rely heavily on the reported comorbidity data to predict risk and associated healthcare costs. Medicare, for example, has been able to estimate the cost that a beneficiary will incur to the government based on their medical history. However, in order for their predictions to be accurate, the coded data must be reliable. On the other hand, coded data do not optimize patient outcomes, educate physicians, or rectify conflicting documentation.

**73. C:** The 21st Century Cures Act Final Rule was established to enable a seamless exchange of electronic health information among multiple healthcare providers without having to obtain authorization or permission from the patient. This would also serve a twofold purpose in encouraging patients and caregivers to take control of the management of their own health because their own healthcare records and results would be more easily accessible to them through various online portals. Additionally, because the Cures Act only applies to physicians and healthcare facilities having an electronic health record (EHR) system, those maintaining paper records are encouraged to abide by information blocking rules by promptly fulfilling a patient's request for medical records.

**74. C:** Due to the volume of patients seen each week, it would be difficult for a physician to recall the specific details of a patient seen more than 48 hours prior. Therefore, in order for records to be accurate and reliable, Medicare advises physicians to complete their documentation within 24–48 hours after a patient is seen. Aside from addendums for unusual circumstances, anything added to a medical record after 48 hours is considered outside the reasonable timeframe.

**75. C:** Prior to 2021, an E/M being leveled based on documentation took into account the history, examination, and MDM involved for a patient. However, effective January 2021, AMA and CMS determined that although an outpatient encounter should include a medically appropriate history and examination, only the documented MDM should be considered during level selection for an outpatient E/M service. In this scenario, because the patient is established and the MDM level is moderate, the E/M level would be 99214.

**76. A:** In order to report CPT code 99242 (office or other outpatient consultation for a new or established patient), a request from another healthcare professional must be on file. The request may be in the form of a prescription, referral, or letter. This code requires a medically appropriate history and/or examination and straightforward medical decision making. When using total time on the date of the encounter for code selection, 20 minutes must be met or exceeded. Additionally, the physician performing the consultation must document their opinion of the patient's condition, illness, and/or injury and return their findings to the physician requesting the consultation. This may be sent electronically, by fax, or through the mail. Consultation CPT codes should not be reported for encounters that occur on the request of a family member.

**77. D:** In this scenario, anemia is coded as the primary diagnosis code. This is because the anemia is the reason for admission and is not associated with the malignancy in the prostate. Instead, it is due to an adverse effect of radiotherapy treatment. ICD-10-CM guidelines give additional guidance in advising not to code T45.1X5– (adverse effect of antineoplastic and immunosuppressive drugs), but to follow the neoplasm code with Y84.2 (radiotherapy as the cause of abnormal reaction of the patient, or of later complication).

**78. A:** Queries must be nonleading, unbiased, legible, grammatically correct, and with no references to reimbursement or cost. In this scenario, the query is compliant with the above requirements and is considered open ended. An open-ended query allows a physician to choose how to best respond to the query. Because of this, a physician may not always provide a diagnosis in line with the documented findings in the chart.

**79. D:** A claim denied due to coordination of benefits indicates that the patient is either not insured with the health plan billed or the patient has additional coverage that should have been billed first. A prior authorization is a request made to an insurance company to take a certain course of treatment. If a request is needed, but not obtained, a payer may deny payment for the services rendered. Timely filing limits are an allowed timeframe given to physicians and facilities to bill for their services. The timeframe varies with each payer, but most often it is 90 days from the date of service. A medical necessity denial indicates that the payer did not agree with the course of treatment rendered by the physician.

**80. D:** The patient financial services (PFS) department will typically have an elaborate understanding of billing rules, such as NCDs and local medical review policies, which both outline the clinical circumstances under which Medicare and Medicare Advantage Plans will render payment on specific procedure codes. On the other hand, medical coders will usually have a thorough knowledge of applying NCCI edits. By working together, the PFS and coding departments can create a healthy revenue cycle and limit the volume of unpaid claims.

**81. B:** The three NCCI PTP edits are 0, 1, and 9. An edit of 0 indicates that billing these two procedures together is not allowed and adding a modifier will not bypass the edit. An edit of 1 indicates that a modifier is allowed on the column 2 procedure, when it is appropriate to do so. The modifiers that can be used to bypass edit 1 include anatomic modifiers (E1–E4, FA, F1–F9, TA, T1–T9, LT, RT, LC, LD, RC, LM, RI), global surgery modifiers (24, 25, 57, 58, 78, 79), and other modifiers (27, 59, 91, XE, XS, XP, XU). Finally, an edit of 9 indicates that an NCCI edit does not apply to the two procedures being paired. In this scenario, aspiration of a joint is referred to in the CPT manual as arthrocentesis. An arthrocentesis of two separate large joints without ultrasound guidance should be reported as 20610, 20610-59. Modifier 59 is used to indicate that two procedures were performed independently of each other and require separate reimbursement.

**82. D:** Medicare Part A provides coverage for inpatient services given in hospitals, including critical access hospitals and skilled nursing facilities, and care rendered in a hospice or home health setting. Although CPT code range 99252–99255 (Inpatient or observation consultation for a new or established patient) does meet the requirements to be covered under Medicare Part A, Medicare opted to no longer pay for consultation services, regardless of the setting they are rendered in. This decision came after an OIG compliance report evaluating the documentation of reported consultations, which found that the requirements to bill these services were not being met. This included the referring physician's request for a consult, a written or verbal request detailing why a consult was needed, and a written report of the consulting physician's findings sent to the referring physician.

**83. D:** Metastasis occurs when cancer cells spread from the tissue or organ they originated in, through the blood or lymph system, and continue to grow in a different tissue or organ. For example, if melanoma, a type of skin cancer, spreads to the lymph nodes, the cancer cells in the lymph nodes are melanoma cells. This new diagnosis would be referred to as lymph metastasis or metastatic lymph nodes and would be coded as C77.– (secondary and unspecified malignant neoplasm of lymph node).

**84. C:** When a procedure or treatment is deemed experimental, the insurance carrier does not view it as medically effective for the condition or illness being treated. In these cases, the next step to obtain payment is to submit an appeal. An appeal is a written letter outlining the reasons why a certain procedure or treatment was medically necessary and the best course of action for this specific patient. Often, including the background of the patient's medical condition (i.e., sustaining a burn in a house fire) and reliable medical studies supporting the procedure will overturn this type of denied claim.

**85. C:** HIPAA-covered entities include health plans, clearinghouses, providers, and business associates. Health plans can be private, but they may also include government programs, such as Medicare, Medicaid, and military and/or veteran health programs. A clearinghouse is an electronic mediator between a provider and a health plan that is responsible for checking data entry errors. A provider may include facilities, such as nursing homes, pharmacies, and clinics, or just a single provider, such as a specialist, psychologist, or dentist. A business associate assists in the activities and functions of a practice that involve the use of PHI, such as an independently contracted medical transcriptionist.

**86. B:** An illness is considered chronic if the expected duration lasts at least 1 year or until the death of the patient. Although stability commonly infers that a condition stays the same, AMA has chosen to define stability in terms of whether or not the patient has achieved their treatment goal. In this scenario, while the diabetes is uncontrolled, or unstable, the physician has decided to focus only on providing comfort. Therefore, the patient has reached their treatment goal, and their condition is considered a stable, chronic illness, which is considered a low-complexity problem.

**87. B:** A charge description master (CDM) is a system file in a hospital or outpatient facility that holds the prices and coding of procedures, drugs, services, and supplies that an entity renders to patients. Maintaining an updated CDM is important in order to ensure compliance with billing practices set forth by CMS, OIG, and other managed care plans; to receive proper reimbursement; to capture unpaid and missing charges; and outline transparent pricing information that the public can access.

**88. B:** Global obstetrical care encompasses antepartum care, delivery services, and postpartum care when rendered by the same physician. It requires that a physician bill just one code for payment at the completion of the patient's postpartum care, to include CPT codes 59400 for a vaginal delivery, 59510 for a Cesarean delivery, 59610 for a vaginal delivery following a previous Cesarean delivery, and 59618 for a Cesarean delivery after an attempted vaginal delivery. For routine prenatal care rendered when a patient's insurance plan only accepts global obstetrical care, use placeholder codes 0500F–0503F (prenatal and postpartum care visit). This indicates that there was an encounter with the patient, but no charges are billed.

**89. A:** According to HHS, if the government declares a public health emergency, PHI may be disclosed to a public health authority "that is authorized by law to collect or receive such information for the purpose of preventing or controlling disease." HIPAA does allow correctional facilities to obtain, without authorization, PHI for the safety of their staff and other inmates and for providing healthcare to the inmate of whom medical records were obtained. For the safety of a child, HIPAA allows disclosure of PHI to law enforcement agencies, including child protective services, without authorization from a legal guardian for a suspected or confirmed case of abuse or neglect.

**90. B:** Encryption turns text, such as PHI, into indecipherable characters that can only be translated when a password or other authentication is provided. Encryption has proven to be a very useful tool in preventing breaches in PHI because hackers are unable to access the data. Additionally, if a device containing PHI has an encryption tool installed, the Office of Civil Rights (OCR) and HHS waive the monetary penalties usually associated with such an incident.

**91. A:** Computer-assisted coding (CAC) is a software application that documents and generates diagnosis codes based on a physician's clinical documentation. CAC is most effective when an encoder is embedded within the CAC software so that the NCCI edits, reimbursement methodologies, and coding guidelines are factored into the code selection. It is also helpful when a facility has fully shifted to an EHR system because CAC is an automatic process.

**92. C:** According to CMS guidelines, if a patient is admitted for inpatient hospital care and is discharged less than 8 hours later on the same date of service, only CPT code range 99221–99223 (initial hospital care, per day, for E/M of a patient) should be reported for the care rendered. Alternately, if the patient was admitted to inpatient hospital care and discharged 8 or more hours later on the same date of service, CPT code range 99234–99236 (inpatient hospital care ... of a patient including admission and discharge on the same date) should be reported.

**93. C:** Amniocentesis is an obstetrical term used to describe an invasive method of determining if a fetus is at risk for chromosomal abnormalities or heart defects. During the procedure, the physician inserts a needle through the maternal abdomen and aspirates amniotic fluid directly from the amniotic sac. By searching "amniocentesis" in the CPT Expert Index, code selection indicates that this procedure is done only with regard to a fetus.

**94. B:** The purpose of the minimum necessary requirement is to ensure that healthcare practices are giving out only the PHI that will satisfy the specific purpose of the request or to carry out a function. For example, an employee may access a patient's intake form and insurance card to verify eligibility and coverage. However, under the minimum necessary requirement, this same employee may not access this patient's medical history, lab results, or related medical records because that information is not necessary to fulfill her job function. Therefore, the minimum necessary requirement would apply to this employee. On the other hand, this requirement does not apply to requests by healthcare providers for the purpose of treatment, patients requesting their own medical records, those whom a patient has authorized to receive medical records, and disclosure as required by law such as in the case of child abuse or neglect.

**95. D:** When a physician deems that additional information should be added to a note after it has already been completed, the physician may add an addendum. An addendum is a clinical entry added to an existing, signed report to provide information that was not available to the physician at the time of entry. Addendums will have their own date, time, and signature line and do not change the existing information in the report. A late entry would be used if the physician knew some clinical information, but unintentionally omitted it from the report and later remembered to add it in. A correction is used to address errors within a report.

**96. A:** Although it is very possible that the cause of the patient's chest pain is a myocardial infarction, it is not documented anywhere else in the patient's chart. Because chest pain can also indicate coronary artery disease with angina or anxiety, a diagnosis of myocardial infarction is not clinically supported. In option B, feelings of numbness may indicate that the patient has neuropathy, and a query may be sent to establish the specificity of the potential condition associated with the diabetes. In option C, because the patient is still receiving chemotherapy treatments, a query may be sent to clarify whether the diagnosis of malignancy is still relevant. In option D, a query may be sent to resolve the conflicting information.

**97. A:** Fraud and abuse both occur when a physician or ancillary staff member submits a false claim. This includes billing for services not rendered, billing for a higher level of service than was actually provided or documented for, and/or ordering unnecessary services. Although they are similar, fraud is committed when there is forethought and intention behind the action, whereas abuse occurs unknowingly. When the fraudulent activity involves a federally funded program, such as Medicare, the result is a violation of the False Claims Act. Finally, waste is an overuse of services or supplies that results in unnecessary costs to the Medicare Program. In this scenario, the physician should have reported only the Cesarean delivery (CPT code 59514). Because this was done in error, the doctor may be charged with healthcare abuse.

**98. B:** For an associated condition that develops after a COVID-19 infection, the condition should be assigned first, followed by the diagnosis of post COVID-19 condition (U09.9). Encounter for follow-up examination after completing treatment (Z09) should not be reported because the patient is receiving ongoing care for the sequelae of the infection. A history of COVID-19 (Z86.16) should also not be reported because U09.9 "excludes 1" Z86.16, indicating that these two conditions should never be reported together. Finally, by verifying the code in the tabular section, persistent cough is coded as R05.3 (chronic cough).

**99. A:** Code 44950 (appendectomy) billed with modifier 50 (bilateral procedure) will get denied under NCCI's MUE. Because there is only one appendix in the human body, the maximum number of units a physician can report is one. Modifier 50 would not apply because there is no opposite, identical structure to remove.

**100. B:** HFpEF, otherwise known as diastolic heart failure, is a condition in which the left ventricle of the heart is unable to fill and pump blood properly. This condition can either be acute, chronic, or both simultaneously. The diagnosis code for HFpEF can be found by locating "failure" in the ICD-10-CM alphabetical index, followed by "heart." If the abbreviation of pEF (preserved ejection fraction) is known, a coder can search that phrase next. If it is unknown, review codes in category I50.-, where the description "heart failure with preserved ejection fraction (HFpEF)" is found under I50.3-.

**101. C:** When a patient is involved in an auto accident, the medical services, supplies, and treatment rendered as a result of the injury are covered under the limits of the automobile's personal injury protection, also known as no-fault insurance. In order to receive reimbursement, healthcare entities must report the claim number of the accident with their charges, which can be obtained by the no-fault insurance carrier, by calling and providing the patient's name and the date of the accident.

**102. B:** The PFS department may reach out to a coder when a claim is denied due to an inappropriate modifier. In this scenario, a double lung transplant does not need modifier 50 appended to it because it is already considered a bilateral procedure. However, the PFS department is not trained in coding or NCCI edits and would therefore not have the expertise to know what should be altered or changed on the claim. On the other hand, they can add the date of the accident to a workers' compensation or no-fault claim, can request retroactive authorization for a procedure, and can write off a balance for noncovered services without permission or clarification from the coding department.

**103. D:** If a definitive diagnosis has been made by the physician, the signs and symptoms normally associated with that disease should not be reported. Chapter 18 of ICD-10-CM contains many symptoms, but not all. In this scenario, weakness (R53.1), dehydration (E86.0), and deconditioning (R53.81) are all symptoms of COVID-19 (U07.1) and pneumonia (J12.82). On the other hand, the patient's advanced age (R54) should be reported as the physician took note of it, and this puts her at a higher risk of developing a severe illness.

**104. D:** Modifier 73 is appended to indicate that an outpatient procedure was terminated by the physician before the start of the procedure, but after surgical preparation, due to extenuating circumstances that threatened the health of the patient. In this scenario, the surgical preparation had begun because the patient was brought to the surgical room. However, the procedure was discontinued prior to the administration of anesthesia and the insertion of a laparoscope. The reason for the procedure, even if not performed, should always be the first-listed diagnosis. In this scenario, because there is a cause-and-effect relationship between the urinary tract infection (N39.0) and the procedure not being carried out, it should be coded as a secondary diagnosis. Additionally, Z53.09 may be assigned as a tertiary code to further explain the circumstances of the encounter.

**105. A:** Administrative safeguards protect PHI from a management perspective. This may include, but is not limited to, an employee receiving the policies and procedures of their employer at the time of hire or deciding who disables a user's information at the time of termination. Physical safeguards prevent the physical removal of PHI and should be appropriate based on factors such as the size and location of an organization. This may include having a security camera or a lock on the server room door. Technical safeguards refer to the security of information systems, such as encryption, firewalls, and internal audits to track employees who access PHI. Although it is recommended to change a password every 60 or 90 days, HIPAA does not outline a password expiration requirement.

**106. A:** Although ICD-10, CPT, and HCPCS level II codes are updated annually with code deletions, additions, and changes, NCDs and LCDs are updated quarterly. In order to keep current with the changes in pricing and coverage, facilities and hospitals should review theirCDM quarterly. Additionally, a CDM audit should be performed on an entity every year in order to ensure that accurate and consistent claims are being submitted and reimbursed appropriately.

**107. B:** On the day a procedure occurs, most physicians will briefly examine and counsel their patient. As a result, an inherent E/M service is included and considered a bundled charge when reported with any procedure code. However, in certain cases in which a physician or other healthcare provider addresses an issue unrelated to the procedure, an E/M service may also be billed. Modifier 25 should be appended on the E/M service to indicate that the illness or disease required additional care not associated with the procedure code.

**108. D:** The diagnosis is always based on the provider's documentation, which in this case would be obesity. Coding guidelines also state that if there is a reportable diagnosis related to weight, "the BMI can be assigned from the documentation of someone other than the patient's provider, such as nursing notes." Although the extracted BMI in this scenario may support a diagnosis of morbid obesity, the provider has only indicated an unspecified obesity. Therefore, only obesity should be reported with the extracted BMI.

**109. B:** When a teaching physician has independently evaluated the patient or was physically present for the critical portions of an exam rendered by a resident and takes part in the management of care, the teaching physician may bill for the care rendered by the resident. However, the teaching physician must implicitly document this in the form of an attestation. An attestation is written proof of what was done. Options A, C, and D are considered unacceptable attestations because it is unclear whether the teaching physician had any physical involvement in the patient's care.

**110. A:** Bundling is a term used to describe two procedures that are inclusive to each other. Unless there is a special circumstance that would allow it, only one CPT code should be reported for both services rendered on the same day. In this scenario, 31231 (nasal endoscopy, diagnostic) is considered a bundled charge of 30801 (ablation, soft tissue of inferior turbinates, any method) since a physician must examine the nose prior to reducing inflammation or removing excessive mucosa by means of ablation.

**111. A:** CPT code 11981 (insertion, drug-delivery implant) is considered mutually exclusive to CPT code 11982 (removal, nonbiodegradable drug delivery implant), meaning that both procedure codes are presumed to never take place at the same anatomical site or at the same time. However, in a scenario in which the patient returns in the same day, both procedures may be billed with modifier 59 appended to the procedure with the expected lower reimbursement rate. This indicates to payers that two procedures were performed independently of each other and require separate reimbursement.

**112. A:** When a condition or illness arises that alters the course of treatment or surgery for a patient, it is known as a complication of care and should be reported. However, some conditions that arise are expected and even considered a normal. In such an instance in which no additional treatment is required, this would not be considered a complication of care. In general, the diagnosis of ileus is often considered an expected outcome of any procedure taking place in the abdominal cavity. At times, a physician may be proactive and perform an ultrasound, electrical stimulation, or administer IV fluids. If this were the case, K91.89 (other postprocedural complications and disorders of digestive system) may be assigned. However, if the physician takes no additional treatment action, report only Z48.815 (encounter for surgical aftercare following surgery on the digestive system) to indicate continued care during the recovery phase.

# How to Overcome Test Anxiety

Just the thought of taking a test is enough to make most people a little nervous. A test is an important event that can have a long-term impact on your future, so it's important to take it seriously and it's natural to feel anxious about performing well. But just because anxiety is normal, that doesn't mean that it's helpful in test taking, or that you should simply accept it as part of your life. Anxiety can have a variety of effects. These effects can be mild, like making you feel slightly nervous, or severe, like blocking your ability to focus or remember even a simple detail.

If you experience test anxiety—whether severe or mild—it's important to know how to beat it. To discover this, first you need to understand what causes test anxiety.

## Causes of Test Anxiety

While we often think of anxiety as an uncontrollable emotional state, it can actually be caused by simple, practical things. One of the most common causes of test anxiety is that a person does not feel adequately prepared for their test. This feeling can be the result of many different issues such as poor study habits or lack of organization, but the most common culprit is time management. Starting to study too late, failing to organize your study time to cover all of the material, or being distracted while you study will mean that you're not well prepared for the test. This may lead to cramming the night before, which will cause you to be physically and mentally exhausted for the test. Poor time management also contributes to feelings of stress, fear, and hopelessness as you realize you are not well prepared but don't know what to do about it.

Other times, test anxiety is not related to your preparation for the test but comes from unresolved fear. This may be a past failure on a test, or poor performance on tests in general. It may come from comparing yourself to others who seem to be performing better or from the stress of living up to expectations. Anxiety may be driven by fears of the future—how failure on this test would affect your educational and career goals. These fears are often completely irrational, but they can still negatively impact your test performance.

## Elements of Test Anxiety

As mentioned earlier, test anxiety is considered to be an emotional state, but it has physical and mental components as well. Sometimes you may not even realize that you are suffering from test anxiety until you notice the physical symptoms. These can include trembling hands, rapid heartbeat, sweating, nausea, and tense muscles. Extreme anxiety may lead to fainting or vomiting. Obviously, any of these symptoms can have a negative impact on testing. It is important to recognize them as soon as they begin to occur so that you can address the problem before it damages your performance.

The mental components of test anxiety include trouble focusing and inability to remember learned information. During a test, your mind is on high alert, which can help you recall information and stay focused for an extended period of time. However, anxiety interferes with your mind's natural processes, causing you to blank out, even on the questions you know well. The strain of testing during anxiety makes it difficult to stay focused, especially on a test that may take several hours. Extreme anxiety can take a huge mental toll, making it difficult not only to recall test information but even to understand the test questions or pull your thoughts together.

# Effects of Test Anxiety

Test anxiety is like a disease—if left untreated, it will get progressively worse. Anxiety leads to poor performance, and this reinforces the feelings of fear and failure, which in turn lead to poor performances on subsequent tests. It can grow from a mild nervousness to a crippling condition. If allowed to progress, test anxiety can have a big impact on your schooling, and consequently on your future.

Test anxiety can spread to other parts of your life. Anxiety on tests can become anxiety in any stressful situation, and blanking on a test can turn into panicking in a job situation. But fortunately, you don't have to let anxiety rule your testing and determine your grades. There are a number of relatively simple steps you can take to move past anxiety and function normally on a test and in the rest of life.

# Physical Steps for Beating Test Anxiety

While test anxiety is a serious problem, the good news is that it can be overcome. It doesn't have to control your ability to think and remember information. While it may take time, you can begin taking steps today to beat anxiety.

Just as your first hint that you may be struggling with anxiety comes from the physical symptoms, the first step to treating it is also physical. Rest is crucial for having a clear, strong mind. If you are tired, it is much easier to give in to anxiety. But if you establish good sleep habits, your body and mind will be ready to perform optimally, without the strain of exhaustion. Additionally, sleeping well helps you to retain information better, so you're more likely to recall the answers when you see the test questions.

Getting good sleep means more than going to bed on time. It's important to allow your brain time to relax. Take study breaks from time to time so it doesn't get overworked, and don't study right before bed. Take time to rest your mind before trying to rest your body, or you may find it difficult to fall asleep.

Along with sleep, other aspects of physical health are important in preparing for a test. Good nutrition is vital for good brain function. Sugary foods and drinks may give a burst of energy but this burst is followed by a crash, both physically and emotionally. Instead, fuel your body with protein and vitamin-rich foods.

Also, drink plenty of water. Dehydration can lead to headaches and exhaustion, especially if your brain is already under stress from the rigors of the test. Particularly if your test is a long one, drink water during the breaks. And if possible, take an energy-boosting snack to eat between sections.

Along with sleep and diet, a third important part of physical health is exercise. Maintaining a steady workout schedule is helpful, but even taking 5-minute study breaks to walk can help get your blood pumping faster and clear your head. Exercise also releases endorphins, which contribute to a positive feeling and can help combat test anxiety.

When you nurture your physical health, you are also contributing to your mental health. If your body is healthy, your mind is much more likely to be healthy as well. So take time to rest, nourish your body with healthy food and water, and get moving as much as possible. Taking these physical steps will make you stronger and more able to take the mental steps necessary to overcome test anxiety.

# Mental Steps for Beating Test Anxiety

Working on the mental side of test anxiety can be more challenging, but as with the physical side, there are clear steps you can take to overcome it. As mentioned earlier, test anxiety often stems from lack of preparation, so the obvious solution is to prepare for the test. Effective studying may be the most important weapon you have for beating test anxiety, but you can and should employ several other mental tools to combat fear.

First, boost your confidence by reminding yourself of past success—tests or projects that you aced. If you're putting as much effort into preparing for this test as you did for those, there's no reason you should expect to fail here. Work hard to prepare; then trust your preparation.

Second, surround yourself with encouraging people. It can be helpful to find a study group, but be sure that the people you're around will encourage a positive attitude. If you spend time with others who are anxious or cynical, this will only contribute to your own anxiety. Look for others who are motivated to study hard from a desire to succeed, not from a fear of failure.

Third, reward yourself. A test is physically and mentally tiring, even without anxiety, and it can be helpful to have something to look forward to. Plan an activity following the test, regardless of the outcome, such as going to a movie or getting ice cream.

When you are taking the test, if you find yourself beginning to feel anxious, remind yourself that you know the material. Visualize successfully completing the test. Then take a few deep, relaxing breaths and return to it. Work through the questions carefully but with confidence, knowing that you are capable of succeeding.

Developing a healthy mental approach to test taking will also aid in other areas of life. Test anxiety affects more than just the actual test—it can be damaging to your mental health and even contribute to depression. It's important to beat test anxiety before it becomes a problem for more than testing.

# Study Strategy

Being prepared for the test is necessary to combat anxiety, but what does being prepared look like? You may study for hours on end and still not feel prepared. What you need is a strategy for test prep. The next few pages outline our recommended steps to help you plan out and conquer the challenge of preparation.

## STEP 1: SCOPE OUT THE TEST

Learn everything you can about the format (multiple choice, essay, etc.) and what will be on the test. Gather any study materials, course outlines, or sample exams that may be available. Not only will this help you to prepare, but knowing what to expect can help to alleviate test anxiety.

## STEP 2: MAP OUT THE MATERIAL

Look through the textbook or study guide and make note of how many chapters or sections it has. Then divide these over the time you have. For example, if a book has 15 chapters and you have five days to study, you need to cover three chapters each day. Even better, if you have the time, leave an extra day at the end for overall review after you have gone through the material in depth.

If time is limited, you may need to prioritize the material. Look through it and make note of which sections you think you already have a good grasp on, and which need review. While you are studying, skim quickly through the familiar sections and take more time on the challenging parts.

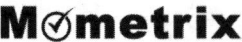

Write out your plan so you don't get lost as you go. Having a written plan also helps you feel more in control of the study, so anxiety is less likely to arise from feeling overwhelmed at the amount to cover.

## STEP 3: GATHER YOUR TOOLS

Decide what study method works best for you. Do you prefer to highlight in the book as you study and then go back over the highlighted portions? Or do you type out notes of the important information? Or is it helpful to make flashcards that you can carry with you? Assemble the pens, index cards, highlighters, post-it notes, and any other materials you may need so you won't be distracted by getting up to find things while you study.

If you're having a hard time retaining the information or organizing your notes, experiment with different methods. For example, try color-coding by subject with colored pens, highlighters, or post-it notes. If you learn better by hearing, try recording yourself reading your notes so you can listen while in the car, working out, or simply sitting at your desk. Ask a friend to quiz you from your flashcards, or try teaching someone the material to solidify it in your mind.

## STEP 4: CREATE YOUR ENVIRONMENT

It's important to avoid distractions while you study. This includes both the obvious distractions like visitors and the subtle distractions like an uncomfortable chair (or a too-comfortable couch that makes you want to fall asleep). Set up the best study environment possible: good lighting and a comfortable work area. If background music helps you focus, you may want to turn it on, but otherwise keep the room quiet. If you are using a computer to take notes, be sure you don't have any other windows open, especially applications like social media, games, or anything else that could distract you. Silence your phone and turn off notifications. Be sure to keep water close by so you stay hydrated while you study (but avoid unhealthy drinks and snacks).

Also, take into account the best time of day to study. Are you freshest first thing in the morning? Try to set aside some time then to work through the material. Is your mind clearer in the afternoon or evening? Schedule your study session then. Another method is to study at the same time of day that you will take the test, so that your brain gets used to working on the material at that time and will be ready to focus at test time.

## STEP 5: STUDY!

Once you have done all the study preparation, it's time to settle into the actual studying. Sit down, take a few moments to settle your mind so you can focus, and begin to follow your study plan. Don't give in to distractions or let yourself procrastinate. This is your time to prepare so you'll be ready to fearlessly approach the test. Make the most of the time and stay focused.

Of course, you don't want to burn out. If you study too long you may find that you're not retaining the information very well. Take regular study breaks. For example, taking five minutes out of every hour to walk briskly, breathing deeply and swinging your arms, can help your mind stay fresh.

As you get to the end of each chapter or section, it's a good idea to do a quick review. Remind yourself of what you learned and work on any difficult parts. When you feel that you've mastered the material, move on to the next part. At the end of your study session, briefly skim through your notes again.

But while review is helpful, cramming last minute is NOT. If at all possible, work ahead so that you won't need to fit all your study into the last day. Cramming overloads your brain with more information than it can process and retain, and your tired mind may struggle to recall even previously learned information when it is overwhelmed with last-minute study. Also, the urgent nature of cramming and the stress placed on your brain contribute to anxiety. You'll be more likely to go to the test feeling unprepared and having trouble thinking clearly.

So don't cram, and don't stay up late before the test, even just to review your notes at a leisurely pace. Your brain needs rest more than it needs to go over the information again. In fact, plan to finish your studies by noon or early afternoon the day before the test. Give your brain the rest of the day to relax or focus on other things, and get a good night's sleep. Then you will be fresh for the test and better able to recall what you've studied.

### STEP 6: TAKE A PRACTICE TEST

Many courses offer sample tests, either online or in the study materials. This is an excellent resource to check whether you have mastered the material, as well as to prepare for the test format and environment.

Check the test format ahead of time: the number of questions, the type (multiple choice, free response, etc.), and the time limit. Then create a plan for working through them. For example, if you have 30 minutes to take a 60-question test, your limit is 30 seconds per question. Spend less time on the questions you know well so that you can take more time on the difficult ones.

If you have time to take several practice tests, take the first one open book, with no time limit. Work through the questions at your own pace and make sure you fully understand them. Gradually work up to taking a test under test conditions: sit at a desk with all study materials put away and set a timer. Pace yourself to make sure you finish the test with time to spare and go back to check your answers if you have time.

After each test, check your answers. On the questions you missed, be sure you understand why you missed them. Did you misread the question (tests can use tricky wording)? Did you forget the information? Or was it something you hadn't learned? Go back and study any shaky areas that the practice tests reveal.

Taking these tests not only helps with your grade, but also aids in combating test anxiety. If you're already used to the test conditions, you're less likely to worry about it, and working through tests until you're scoring well gives you a confidence boost. Go through the practice tests until you feel comfortable, and then you can go into the test knowing that you're ready for it.

## Test Tips

On test day, you should be confident, knowing that you've prepared well and are ready to answer the questions. But aside from preparation, there are several test day strategies you can employ to maximize your performance.

First, as stated before, get a good night's sleep the night before the test (and for several nights before that, if possible). Go into the test with a fresh, alert mind rather than staying up late to study.

Try not to change too much about your normal routine on the day of the test. It's important to eat a nutritious breakfast, but if you normally don't eat breakfast at all, consider eating just a protein bar. If you're a coffee drinker, go ahead and have your normal coffee. Just make sure you time it so that the caffeine doesn't wear off right in the middle of your test. Avoid sugary beverages, and drink enough water to stay hydrated but not so much that you need a restroom break 10 minutes into the test. If your test isn't first thing in the morning, consider going for a walk or doing a light workout before the test to get your blood flowing.

Allow yourself enough time to get ready, and leave for the test with plenty of time to spare so you won't have the anxiety of scrambling to arrive in time. Another reason to be early is to select a good seat. It's helpful to sit away from doors and windows, which can be distracting. Find a good seat, get out your supplies, and settle your mind before the test begins.

When the test begins, start by going over the instructions carefully, even if you already know what to expect. Make sure you avoid any careless mistakes by following the directions.

Then begin working through the questions, pacing yourself as you've practiced. If you're not sure on an answer, don't spend too much time on it, and don't let it shake your confidence. Either skip it and come back later, or eliminate as many wrong answers as possible and guess among the remaining ones. Don't dwell on these questions as you continue—put them out of your mind and focus on what lies ahead.

Be sure to read all of the answer choices, even if you're sure the first one is the right answer. Sometimes you'll find a better one if you keep reading. But don't second-guess yourself if you do immediately know the answer. Your gut instinct is usually right. Don't let test anxiety rob you of the information you know.

If you have time at the end of the test (and if the test format allows), go back and review your answers. Be cautious about changing any, since your first instinct tends to be correct, but make sure you didn't misread any of the questions or accidentally mark the wrong answer choice. Look over any you skipped and make an educated guess.

At the end, leave the test feeling confident. You've done your best, so don't waste time worrying about your performance or wishing you could change anything. Instead, celebrate the successful completion of this test. And finally, use this test to learn how to deal with anxiety even better next time.

> **Review Video: Test Anxiety**
> Visit mometrix.com/academy and enter code: 100340

## Important Qualification

Not all anxiety is created equal. If your test anxiety is causing major issues in your life beyond the classroom or testing center, or if you are experiencing troubling physical symptoms related to your anxiety, it may be a sign of a serious physiological or psychological condition. If this sounds like your situation, we strongly encourage you to seek professional help.

# Additional Bonus Material

Due to our efforts to try to keep this book to a manageable length, we've created a link that will give you access to all of your additional bonus material:

**mometrix.com/bonus948/certcodeasso**